The Complete Idiot's Command Reference

Medical Super Sites

Make these sites your first stops for medical information on the Web. Visit them all, and bookmark your favorites so you can refer to them often. (For information about each site, see Chapter 4, "How to Evaluate a Medical Site.")

Adam.com	`http://www.adam.com`
allHealth from iVillage	`http://www.allhealth.com`
drkoop.com	`http://drkoop.com`
Hardin Meta Directory of Internet Health Sources	`http://www.lib.uiowa.edu/ hardin/md/index.html`
HealthAnswers	`http://healthanswers.com`
HealthAtoZ	`http://www.healthatoz.com`
HealthCentral	`www.healthcentral.com`
Healthfinder	`http://www.healthfinder.gov`
HealthWeb	`http://healthweb.org`
InteliHealth	`http://www.intelihealth.com`
LaurusHealth	`http://www.laurushealth.com`
Mayo Clinic Health Oasis	`http://www.mayohealth.org`
Mediconsult	`http://www.mediconsult.com`
MEDLINE	`http://igm.nlm.nih.gov`
New York Online Access to Health (NOAH)	`http://www.noah.cuny.edu`
OnHealth	`http://onhealth.com`
StayHealthy.com	`http://www.stayhealthy.com`
WebMDHealth	`http://my.webmd.com`
WellnessWeb	`http://wellweb.com`

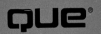

cut here

The PILOT Method

How do you know if you've found a credible medical Web site? The PILOT Method will help you evaluate it.

P Purpose

If the site has a mission statement, read it. If not, read the home page and analyze the site's purpose. Does it inform and educate? Or is it designed to persuade, sell, outrage, or entertain?

I Information

Truly useful medical Web sites offer valuable information and emphasize facts rather than opinion and testimonials. If the site is selling *anything*, ask yourself if that influences the content.

L Links

The best sites want to inform you and are happy to recommend additional Web sites to further your knowledge in that topic or related topics. The best links are rated or reviewed.

O Originator

Who is responsible for the information? Best bets for sound medical information are medical societies, consumer-advocacy groups, well-known hospitals, and government- and university-sponsored sites.

T Timeliness

Medical information is only useful if it is current. Look for sites that update frequently.

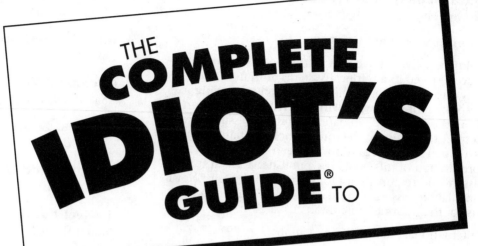

THE

COMPLETE
IDIOT'S
GUIDE® TO

Online Medical
Resources

DISCARDED
from
New Hanover County Public Library

by Joan Price

que®

A Division of Macmillan USA
201 W. 103rd Street, Indianapolis, IN 46290

The Complete Idiot's Guide to Online Medical Resources

Copyright © 2000 by Que®

International Standard Book Number: 0-7897-2297-6

Library of Congress Catalog Card Number: 99-067315

Printed in the United States of America

First Printing: March 2000

02 01 00   4   3   2   1

Trademarks

Warning and Disclaimer

Associate Publisher
Greg Wiegand

Acquisitions Editor
Angelina Ward

Development Editor
Sarah Robbins

Technical Editor
Doug Dafforn

Managing Editor
Thomas F. Hayes

Project Editor
Karen S. Shields

Copy Editor
Molly Schaller

Indexer
Sheila Schroeder

Proofreader
Jeanne Clark

Illustrator
Judd Winick

Team Coordinator
Sharry Gregory

Interior Designer
Nathan Clement

Cover Designer
Michael Freeland

Copywriter
Eric Borgert

Editorial Assistant
Angela Boley

Production
Lisa England

Contents at a Glance

Contents

20 Cancer 251

21 Diabetes 269

22 Depression 279

Foreword

When Joan Price and Shannon Entin wrote *The Complete Idiot's Guide to Online Health and Fitness*, I was elated that finally consumers could find an accurate, practical, and simple guide to using the Internet for health and fitness information. Now Joan Price has taken readers to the next step—showing them how to evaluate online medical information. Thanks to Joan, consumers have a smart, friendly, step-by-step guide to maneuvering through the quagmire of medical misinformation to find solid, credible resources.

I battle medical misunderstanding daily. Listeners to my radio program and readers of HealthCentral.com are always saying to me, "Dr. Edell, I read about this new cancer cure on the Internet," or "I don't like to go to doctors, so I went to a Web site on my disease and I ordered these herbs." Sometimes I feel like my readers and listeners are drowning in a sea of misinformation, rumor, and fraud. It's not their fault—they never went to medical school. How are they going to know whether they're reading facts or fantasies? This book is their crash course in evaluating the medical information they read online.

Thank you, Joan, for making my job easier!

—Dean Edell, M.D., media medical reporter and author of *Eat, Drink & Be Merry* (Harper Collins, 1999)

http://healthcentral.com

Dedication

First, I'd like to thank you, the reader, for picking up this book, seeing the value in it, and letting it become your guide on this marvelous journey.

I am indebted to the many medical experts who advised me and the Web site content providers who make the World Wide Web such an enriching, educational experience. Many of you are quoted or cited in the book, others offered wisdom behind the scenes, and I thank you all. Thanks also to Chris Hendel for his invaluable research assistance and to Dean Edell, M.D., whose clear and feisty explanations stretch my knowledge constantly.

Thank you, Shannon Entin, co-author of my first book in this series, *The Complete Idiot's Guide to Online Health and Fitness,* and the founder/publisher/editor extraordinaire of *Fitness Link*. Your influence sparkles on the pages of this book, too!

Thanks to the amazing team at Macmillan, whose talents and dedication to excellence brought out the best in this book. Special thanks to Angelina Ward, acquisitions editor, for her unique level of support.

Thanks to my dear friends for the joy and insights they bring to my life (and for making sure I leave my computer once in a while!). Thank you, Dan Goldes, for almost two decades of friendship and understanding. Thank you, Chris Overholt, for being my sister and cheerleader. Thank you, John Martin, for always listening and believing in me. And thank you, Joshua Boneh, for all the dances—they keep me whole and happy.

Tell Us What You Think!

As the reader of this book, *you* are our most important critic and commentator. We value your opinion and want to know what we're doing right, what we could do better, what areas you'd like to see us publish in, and any other words of wisdom you're willing to pass our way.

As an Associate Publisher for Que, I welcome your comments. You can fax, email, or write me directly to let me know what you did or didn't like about this book—as well as what we can do to make our books stronger.

Please note that I cannot help you with technical problems related to the topic of this book, and that due to the high volume of mail I receive, I might not be able to reply to every message.

When you write, please be sure to include this book's title and author as well as your name and phone or fax number. I will carefully review your comments and share them with the author and editors who worked on the book.

Fax: 317-581-4666

Email: consumer@mcp.com

Mail: Greg Wiegand,
          Associate Publisher
          Que
          201 West 103rd Street
          Indianapolis, IN 46290 USA

Introduction

Mark Twain didn't believe in reading medical information. "You could die of a misprint," he wrote. Imagine what he'd say about the craziness people read on the Internet!

Estimates are that 35.5 million adults in the United States will search for medical information online in the year 2000, five times as many surfers as five years earlier. These medical-information seekers will find huge variations in quality, from top-quality sources of reliable information to scummy scams designed to rob you blind.

These surfers will encounter hundreds of thousands of sites somewhere between those two extremes. The sites might have some valid information hidden under a blanket of misinformation. Or they might promote an unproven treatment zealously, believing it to be the almighty cure. Or their agenda might be to sell you products rather than to inform you. It's like wandering blindly through a maze!

Enter the guide dog, relentlessly sniffing out the good, the bad, the ugly, and the just plain silly. This book points you to outstanding Web sites covering a variety of medical topics, including some fresh ones that even experienced surfers probably don't know.

More important, this book teaches you how to find the information you seek on your own and how to evaluate the Web sites you find on the journey. You learn to read the Information Superhighway road map and drive yourself to your destination, steering away from scams, frauds, and misleading claims and advice. You learn to read the signs that tell you which sites are worth long visits.

How to Use This Book

You don't have to read every chapter—though, of course, I wish you would!—or go in order. This book is organized into five parts. Even if you skip around, definitely read all of Part 1 first, because it has general information and guidelines that apply to whatever medical information you seek online.

Part 1, "Getting Started, Getting Savvy," shows you where to start to find and evaluate the major medical sites on the World Wide Web.

Part 2, "You and Your Medical Care," shows you how to use the Internet for your own personal medical needs: choosing health care, buying medical supplies, and making your physician your partner.

Part 3, "Staying Well," helps you stay healthy with chapters focusing on the health and wellness concerns of women, men, and children, with a special chapter on sexuality.

Part 4, "Getting Well: Surgery, Drugs, and Alternatives," guides you toward solid information about treatments you might be considering, and away from ads and scams. The chapter on addictions shows you how the Internet can be a partner in recovery.

Part 5, "Diseases and Disorders," shows you where to find the best information about 10 specific conditions: allergies and asthma, Alzheimer's disease, arthritis, back pain, cancer, diabetes, depression, heart disease, HIV/AIDS, and osteoporosis.

Extras

You'll see these tips, cautions, and distinguished sites in boxes splashed throughout the book:

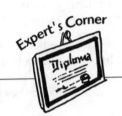

Expert's Corner

Quotes from experts in different health fields offering tips, comments, and cautions about getting accurate information.

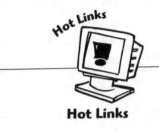

Hot Links

Unique Web sites that are worth a visit.

Support Groups

Newsgroups, mailing lists, chats, bulletin boards, and special Web sites to help you find the online support you need.

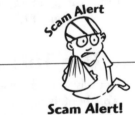

Scam Alert!

Warnings for avoiding frauds, rip-offs, and misleading advice.

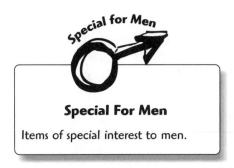

Special For Men

Items of special interest to men.

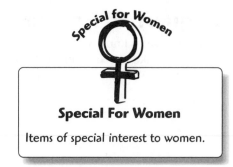

Special For Women

Items of special interest to women.

Disclaimer

Of course, this book and the Web sites mentioned in it are not substitutes for medical advice and should not be used as diagnosis, prescription, or treatment. But you knew that.

Special Thanks

First, I'd like to thank you, the reader, for picking up this book, seeing the value in it, and letting it become your guide on this marvelous journey.

I am indebted to the many medical experts who advised me, and to the Web site content providers who make the World Wide Web such a rich, educational experience. Many of you are quoted or cited in the book, others offered wisdom behind the scenes, and I thank you all. Thanks also to Chris Hendel for his invaluable research assistance and to Dean Edell, M.D., whose clear and feisty explanations stretch my knowledge constantly.

Thank you, Shannon Entin, co-author of my first book in this series, *The Complete Idiot's Guide to Online Health & Fitness,* and the founder/publisher/editor extraordinaire of Fitness Link. Your influence sparkles on the pages of this book, too!

Thanks to the amazing team at Macmillan, whose talents and dedication to excellence brought out the best in this book. Special thanks to Angelina Ward, acquisitions editor, for her unique level of support.

Thanks to my dear friends for the joy and insights they bring to my life (and for making sure I leave my computer once in a while!). Thank you, Dan Goldes, for almost two decades of friendship and understanding. Thank you, Chris Overholt, for being my sister and cheerleader. Thank you, John Martin, for always listening and believing in me. And thank you, Joshua Boneh, for all the dances—they keep me whole and happy.

Request to Readers

I'd love to know what you liked about this book and which Web sites and topics you'd like to see included in future editions of this book or new *Complete Idiot's Guides*. You can email me personally at jprice@sonic.net.

Part 1
Getting Started, Getting Savvy

The Internet is your ticket to valuable, in-depth, timely medical information, found in the privacy of your own home and with the ease of a mouse click. But where do you start? And how do you sift the quality information from the abundance of quackery and foolishness online?

The chapters in Part 1 steer you around the tricky curves on the Information Superhighway by showing you the landmarks of credible medical sites and introducing you to some of the best ones. You learn how to evaluate medical Web sites so you recognize the credible sites and don't get snookered by the scams, hard sells, and malarkey that flourish online.

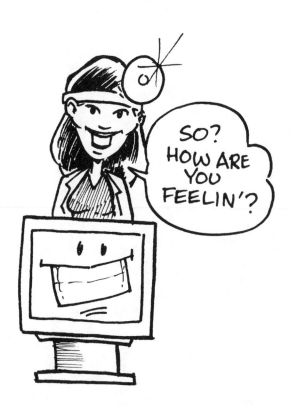

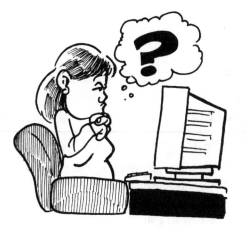

Chapter 1

What Can You Learn Online?

In This Chapter

➤ Ways to use online medical information

➤ Ways *not* to use online medical information

➤ Getting answers to your personal medical questions online

➤ Finding support on the Internet

35.5 million American adults are searching for medical information in the year 2000. If you are one of them, you're in search of credible, reliable sites, and you might be apprehensive about how to find and evaluate them.

This chapter gives you an overview of what you're likely to find, and the benefits and pitfalls of getting medical information on the World Wide Web.

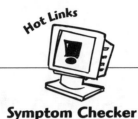

Symptom Checker

`http://onhealth.com/ch1/resource/symptomchecker/index.asp`

You have an ache, pain, or other physical discomfort. Do you need to get medical help? This interactive symptom checker from *Harvard Medical School Family Health Guide* walks you through a series of yes/no questions to determine possible causes, home remedies (when appropriate), and when to call your doctor. This site does not diagnose—it presents several possibilities that fit your symptoms, and alerts you if the symptoms indicate that you should stop surfing and call your doc.

Managing Your Personal Health Care

First, an important caveat: The Internet should never be used as a substitute for live medical attention. Please read that sentence again, commit it to memory, and whisper it to yourself as you surf medical sites.

In particular, information you read on the Internet should never be used to diagnose or treat an illness or condition, prescribe medications (see Chapter 14, "Medications and Supplements," for a convincing argument), or replace a medical examination.

So why all the hullabaloo about medical sites, if you can't even save the cost of a doctor's visit by reading them?

The reputable medical sites on the World Wide Web are the best tools for patient empowerment that the world has seen. Now that's a grandiose statement, granted, but think about it. For the first time in history, health-care consumers have unlimited access to medical information. You can take charge of your personal health care by making the most of the amazing resources available to you.

The following are some examples of what you can learn from medical sites:

➤ Your doctor diagnoses a disease. Look it up on the Web, and you'll find hundreds—maybe thousands—of sites with information about that disease.

➤ You're scheduled for a routine exam. Find out why it's done, what to expect, and what the results mean.

➤ You are considering surgery. Read about the procedure, the reasons for doing it, expected outcome, risks, and costs, and view illustrations.

➤ Keep an online record of your appointments, tests, and prescriptions.

➤ Learn what lifestyle choices help to prevent disease, and adjust your diet, physical activity, and stress for best results.

➤ Keep abreast of the latest health developments and educate yourself about medical topics in the news.

➤ Join motivating support groups to create a community with others who are going through a similar health experience.

➤ Become an educated patient and your physician's partner by supplementing what he or she tells you with information from reputable sites. Read the same medical journals your doctor reads, if you wish!

That's just the beginning of how you can use the medical resources on the Internet!

Look for Disclaimers

Never use the Internet as a substitute for live medical attention. (Are you getting tired of hearing that? And this is just Chapter 1!) If you feel a lump in some body part that didn't used to have one, have chest pains, wonder if St. John's Wort would lift your severe depression, or if your child is crying from an earache, do not use the Internet instead of seeking the help of a live health professional.

Be particularly wary of sites that do not offer the above advice. Reputable sites will post a statement such as the following excerpt from the disclaimer from healthAtoZ.com (http://www.healthatoz.com):

> "All information provided on this site, particularly any information relating to specific medical conditions, health care, preventive care, and healthy lifestyles, is presented for general informational purposes only. It should not be considered complete or exhaustive and does not cover all disorders or conditions or their treatment, nor all health-related issues.

> "The information provided on HealthAtoZ is not intended as a substitute for the advice provided by your own physician or health care provider, and may not necessarily take your individual health situation into account. You should not use the information on HealthAtoZ as a means of diagnosing a health problem or disease, or as a means of determining treatment. You should also not use the information on HealthAtoZ as a substitute for professional medical advice when deciding on any health-related regimen, including diet or exercise. You should always consult a [sic] your own licensed health care provider for these purposes, or for any specific, individual medical advice."

Here's how HealthCentral (http://www.healthcentral.com) deals with the same issue:

"The information provided by HealthCentral.com is for educational and entertainment purposes only and should not be interpreted as a recommendation for a specific treatment plan, product, or course of action. HealthCentral.com does not provide specific medical advice, and is not engaged in providing medical or professional services. Use of HealthCentral.com does not replace medical consultations with a qualified health or medical professional to meet the health and medical needs of yourself or a loved one. In addition, while HealthCentral.com frequently updates its contents, medical information changes rapidly and therefore, some information may be out of date. Please check with a physician or health professional if you suspect you are ill."

Realize that disclaimers such as the above should not make you wary that the information is suspect—quite the contrary. The more credible the site is, the more likely that it will warn you not to diagnose or treat your problem using the site content.

On the other hand, if a site claims to be able to diagnose a medical condition or prescribe medication or other treatment, lace up your virtual running shoes and get out of there.

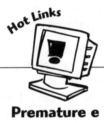

Hot Links

Premature e

http://www.prematuree.com

"Anonymous answers to life's embarrassing questions"—this is definitely a weird site! If you've always wondered about pubic lice, flatulence, or why those red boils form on your buttock cheeks—plus many topics that can't be described in this G-rated book—this is the place to find the answer.

In Search of a Second Opinion

You've agreed that you won't use the Internet to diagnose your medical condition, right? You can still expand your understanding of possible diagnoses while you're waiting for the tests to come back. After you have a diagnosis, you can learn more about what that means, and supplement the information your doctor gave you with responsible online information. If you have an Internet-savvy physician (don't we wish they all were?), he or she might recommend some sites for more information.

Some sites let you "talk" to a doctor. Remember, the cyberdoc is *not* diagnosing or treating your condition, simply offering additional information. This will not be earth-shaking information that sends you running to change your treatment—reputable online docs know that they cannot make these recommendations without examining you and knowing your medical history. But if you're three weeks from your next doctor's appointment and you have a factual question, why not see if you can get your answer online? The following sites help you do it. (All are free unless otherwise noted.)

America's Doctor

http://www.americasdoctor.com

"Real Questions. Real Doctors. Real Time. 24 Hours a Day." You type in your question (it can't be an emergency situation) and wait until a doctor comes online to chat with you. You are told how many people are ahead of you (but no estimate of how long that might take). As you wait, you're free to explore the site, which is full of information, support, and scheduled chats led by experts on a variety of medical topics.

Your Family Doctor

http://www.consult.iperweb.com

Get a confidential "virtual medical consultation" by email. You can read plenty of free content on the site, but the personal consultation is user-supported: Regular consultations (response within 5 business days) are $15; "Sprint" consultations (response within 2 business days) are $25.

Ask the Doctors

http://www.flora.org/ask-doctor/

Email your personal medical question, and it is distributed confidentially to volunteer participating doctors (see Figure 1.1). Those who answer post their responses to the site (without identifying you), and you can read their answers.

Ask the Doctors!

http://www.askthedrs.com

"Real answers from real physicians." Submit your question, and get an answer back by email from a physician. This is a free service if you don't mind waiting for your answer. Pay $12.95 for a reply within 48 hours.

Ask the Tooth Doctor

http://www.askthetoothdoctor.com

Dr. Jack Newton is a cyberdentist who answers your dental questions for free.
Dr. Newton has a hospital-based dental practice at The Ottawa Hospital, in Ottawa, Canada.

11

Figure 1.1

Ask the Doctors lets you ask personal medical questions and read physicians' answers.

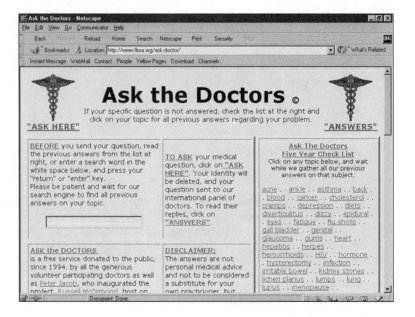

BestDoctors.com

http://www.bestdoctors.com

You have to join (it's free) to participate. After you register, click **The Doctor Is In** to send a question. A physician will email you a response. You can also take part in live online community events.

Under the Microscope: Researching Conditions and Decisions

One of the major ways that the Internet is revolutionizing health care is by permitting patients to take charge of researching their own medical conditions. Rather than the clueless patients of the past, devoid of any medical knowledge, we now arrive at the doctor's office with our minds full of information and our arms full of printouts.

The problem is making sure our minds and arms aren't full of *misinformation*. As you search the Internet for medical information, don't mentally or physically download everything you read. There's too much of it, and a sizable proportion is bound to be inaccurate and/or useless. Yes, there are treasures on the Web, but there's also a lot of trash.

You're more likely to find what you're looking for if you have a plan. First, identify your needs and goals. You wouldn't make a doctor's appointment without knowing what you want to accomplish, whether it's evaluating a health condition, diagnosing a symptom, or curing an ache, pain, or wheeze. Likewise, although you could spend weeks just browsing one medical site after another and gathering intriguing bits of information like you sample the tasters at Costco, the process works better if you know what you're looking for and set your sights (and sites) in that direction.

Your best guide to medical information is your own health professional who knows your medical history firsthand. Make your own physician your ally, not your adversary, in your search for information.

Start by making notes on the information your doctor has already given you, including any pamphlets or other handouts. If possible, phone your doctor and tell him or her that you're searching for information online. If your physician is computer savvy, he or she can tell you about some reliable sites to start with, and some creepy ones to avoid. (See Chapter 7, "You and Your Doc: A Partnership," for much more about how to work with your doctor toward common goals.)

Researching: What's Out There?

The whole world of medicine is available with a few keyboard clicks. You can find information on any disease, however rare. You can read original studies, expert interpretations of those studies, pros and cons of treatments, breaking news about medications—you want it, you can find it.

Where you find it is a big clue about how reliable the information is. This book aims to point you to the best sites, steer you away from the scummy ones, and help you tell the difference. Make these *your* goals, too.

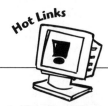

Search Engine Showdown

http://www.notess.com/search

The Search Engine Showdown is a great place to learn about search engines. It offers a chart that compares search capabilities, reviews that tell you the engine's strengths and weaknesses, and tips to make the most of your search. This site covers traditional search engines, as well as "meta" searches, newsgroup searches, and mailing list searches. Read about strategies to help you search the Web effectively, and find links to even more tools.

.Com Versus .Org?

You can get some illuminating information just by reading the extension at the end of the domain name. The domain name follows the "@" sign in an Internet address. The extension comes after the domain name and starts with a "." (Your English teacher called this a "period," but in computer talk, it's a "dot.")

Here's what you can learn about the site's identity just by reading the extension:

➤ **.com** Commercial site

➤ **.edu** Educational site from a four-year college or university

➤ **.gov** U.S. federal government site, which often provides top-quality health information

➤ **.int** Organizations established by international treaty

➤ **.mil** The U.S. military

➤ **.net** Network provider

➤ **.org** Organization or society, often not-for-profit

Many of the best medical sites are government, organization, and education sites. The government (.gov) spends your tax dollars wisely (this time!) with consumer information that saves you money and protects your health. The medical associations and societies (.org) often have superb sites with patient information about their specialties. Some of the top universities and medical schools (.edu) have Web sites with excellent medical content.

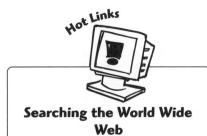

Searching the World Wide Web

http://www.lib.berkeley.edu/ TeachingLib/Guides/Internet/ Strategies.html.

The University of California at Berkeley offers an excellent guide to analyzing your topic, choosing search tools, and using search strategies.

Don't discount the commercial sites, though—some are splendid. The best have a mission to present top-notch public information, such as the .com sites recommended in this book. Most commercial sites, however, aim their content at promoting sales, and are therefore unreliable sources of medical information. Use the PILOT Method in Chapter 4, "How to Evaluate a Medical Site," to assess this.

The .net designation might be the sign of a personal page. The person's Internet service provider provides the home page.

Personal Pages

Web surfer, beware! *Anyone* can put a Web site on the World Wide Web. Publishing a Web site with your own pictures, personal opinions, and tidbits of information is fun, inexpensive (sometimes free), and relatively simple. You don't need a lot of technical know-how, and you certainly don't need to be an "expert" in anything, to put up a Web site. And no one stops shady characters from claiming expertise they don't have, pretending to be doctors, inventing testimonials for their products, or indulging in any other fantasy at the unwary consumer's expense.

As you search for valuable medical information on the Web, you're likely to come across many personal Web pages devoted to miracle cures, weird treatments, and half-cooked advice, in addition to well-meaning, self-proclaimed "experts" who want to give you unfounded and/or unresearched advice. Some of these are really cheesy. Others look like authentic information, but aren't.

A precious few share genuinely helpful information. These are people who researched a topic carefully and want to save you doing all the work yourself. A few of those are mentioned in this book.

Comparing Information

Don't get all your information from one site. A good bet is to compare information about your topic of choice on several of the "Medical Super Sites" recommended in Chapter 4. See how the same basic content is repeated from site to site, and how a topic is treated differently. There might be a different focus, or one site might go more in depth, or some late-breaking news might be prominent on one site.

Then compare the information you found on the sites you know to be reliable with the content on sites you find on your own. If the information is drastically different, treat the off-beat site with unusual information with a healthy dose of skepticism.

If the content on any site is truly unique, tread as cautiously as if you were walking barefoot on broken glass. Beware especially of a site that identifies a "cure" that the major medical sites don't mention—especially if it's selling that "cure"! (Read more about how to identify scam sites in Chapter 3, "Medical Minefield: Watching Where You Step.")

Getting Support

The Internet shines as a pathway to finding a community of people who are going through a health experience similar to yours. You can join email lists, post and read messages on bulletin boards, and ask questions on online chat events.

Many of the Medical Super Sites described in Chapter 4 offer terrific online support groups, and more are mentioned in the chapters about specific diseases. In addition, you can explore sites that specialize in helping you find support resources.

Finding and Using Mailing Lists

Skin cancer? Seasonal affective disorder? Sports injuries? Irritable bowel syndrome? If you're looking for animated and varied discussions on any topic whatsoever, check

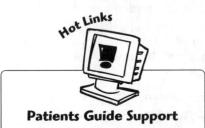

Patients Guide Support

`http://www3.bc.sympatico.ca/`
`me/patientsguide/support.htm`

What are mailing lists, newsgroups, forums, and chats? Are there search engines for finding these? Read brief descriptions of what these are, how they work, and how to get involved with them.

out private *mailing lists* on the Internet. Topics cover everything from acne to Zoloft. The subscribers are passionate and well-informed. To subscribe to a mailing list, send an email message to a subscription address. You have to follow the list's instructions for specifics—each list has a different subscription procedure. Then you receive all the messages posted each day on the list's topic. Be prepared for plenty of email!

Mailing lists can be *moderated* or *unmoderated*. We recommend a moderated list, meaning there is a person who reads every message and forwards only the relevant posts. This cuts down on email traffic, eliminates duplicate topic postings, prevents spam, and keeps the conversation on track. In an unmoderated list, you might find yourself sifting through email hoaxes ("warnings" about computer viruses or "evidence" that certain foods are harmful for you) or personal emails from other members that should have been exchanged off the list.

The following Web sites can help you find mailing lists on any topic:

➤ Liszt, `http://www.liszt.com`

➤ Publicly Accessible Mailing Lists, `http://www.neosoft.com/internet/paml`

➤ Tile.net, `http://www.tile.net/lists/`

➤ CataList, `http://www.1-soft.com/catalist.html`

➤ ONElist, `http://www.onelist.com`

➤ Topica, `http://www.topica.com`

Approach with Caution!

Use caution when discussing any private issues with strangers over the Internet. You don't know who these people are or how they might use your personal information. Be aware that all messages you post—to a mailing list, newsgroup, message board, and sometimes even chat—are archived and kept on the Internet indefinitely. Visit a site like Deja.com and notice how people's posts are readily available for the searching. We advise not using your real name, or at least sticking to first names, and never giving out your address or phone number.

Finding and Using Newsgroups

Newsgroups, often referred to by the technical name *Usenet*, are typically unmoderated and less focused than mailing lists. Messages are posted to an Usenet site and you need to revisit the site day after day to read new postings.

Newsgroups are not on the Web. They have their own interface and you need software called a *newsreader* to access them. Most browsers come with a newsreader (such as Microsoft's Outlook Express or Netscape's Messenger) that enables you to search through the thousands of newsgroups available. You don't subscribe to a newsgroup as you do a mailing list, so participants come and go more often than they do in mailing lists.

Some newsgroups have a core group of participants that are extremely active and helpful, which makes that newsgroup a great place to go to find a real, live person who can answer your question. If you're just looking for an answer to a specific question, and you don't want to join a mailing list and discuss the topic on a regular basis, newsgroups offer an alternative. For example, let's say you read about a new herbal remedy in a magazine and you'd like to find out more from someone who's actually used it. You might visit the misc.health.alternative newsgroup and pose your question. It's likely that someone participating in the newsgroup can tell you whether the herb is useful, has side effects, or is a gimmick.

The following Web sites can help you find newsgroups on any topic:

➤ Deja.com, http://www.deja.com

➤ Tile.net, http://www.tile.net/news

Finding and Using Message Boards

Message boards, also known as *bulletin boards* and *forums*, are similar to newsgroups, but they are typically much smaller and more tightly focused on a single topic than newsgroups are. Message boards are located on Web sites, so they are easy to access—just find a good message board, bookmark it, and visit it regularly to post your messages or respond to others. One caveat—message boards are often unmoderated, which allows for lots of spam, advertising, and unrelated conversation. Search for message boards on the Web at Forum One, http://www.forumone.com.

If you are a member of an online service such as America Online or CompuServe, these services offer tons of message boards that are not available on the Web. Just do a standard keyword search on your topic of interest and the online service points you to relevant message boards.

The following sites help you find message boards about specific topics.

Support-Group.com

http://www.support-group.com

Do you wish you had people to talk to about migraines, alopecia, binge eating, restless leg syndrome, or another health concern? Support-Group.com has searched the

Internet for bulletin boards, chats, organizations, and support sites. Choose from 200 bulletin boards and thousands of links on topics from Aarskog Syndrome to Xeroderma Pigmentosum (see Figure 1.2).

Figure 1.2

Support-Group.com lists more than 200 message boards.

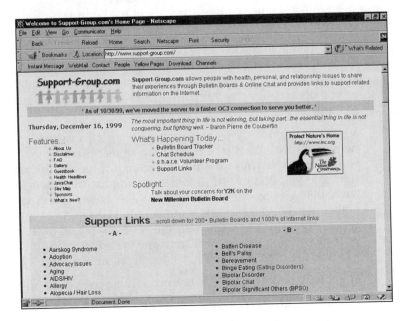

HealthBoards.com

`http://www.healthboards.com`

Connecting with others who have similar medical concerns can help you relate, learn, and cope. HealthBoards.com offers over 800 bulletin boards covering specific health topics on which you can ask questions and discuss medical issues.

Finding and Using Chat Rooms

Chat rooms are areas you can go to "talk" in real time with others on the Internet. You type in your message using your Web browser or chat software and it is instantly relayed to all others in your chat room. And you receive instant responses! It's fun, and it's easy.

More and more Web sites are offering chat rooms—some rooms are open all the time, so you can chat anytime there is someone else in the room. Others have scheduled chat times and topics and even experts and celebrities to answer your questions. The nature of chat doesn't allow for in-depth discussions, but it's a great place to ask questions, make friends, and gain support.

Here's the lowdown on how to chat:

➤ Online services (such as America Online, CompuServe, and Prodigy) offer the easiest access to chat rooms covering hundreds of topics. No special software is needed—just visit the health area of these online services and you can easily find chat rooms that cater to a topic you are interested in.

➤ There are various software programs that enable you to chat over the Internet without using an online service. One such program is called IRC (Internet Relay Chat), `http://www.mirc.com`. Just download the software, install it on your computer, and then use the Liszt site at `http://liszt.com/chat/` to search through more than 37,000 chat rooms, or channels.

➤ Web-based chats work through your standard browser. Just like a bulletin board, you visit the chat Web site, log in, and start chatting. Web-based chat rooms are typically slower and less popular than IRC or online service chats.

Just for Fun

Most of the sites in this book are super serious—you don't want to get your medical information from a comedian. But you might enjoy a little medical humor now and then, and these sites offer giggles, guffaws, and groans.

Diet, Health, and Fitness Cartoons

`http://www.glasbergen.com/fit.html`

Doctor to patient: "To prevent a heart attack, take one aspirin every day. Take it out for a jog, then take it to the gym, then take it for a bike ride…" Cartoonist Randy Glasbergen's health, fitness, and diet cartoons are clever (see Figure 1.3). After you scroll through the cartoons, keep clicking the list at the end—some of the best ones are there.

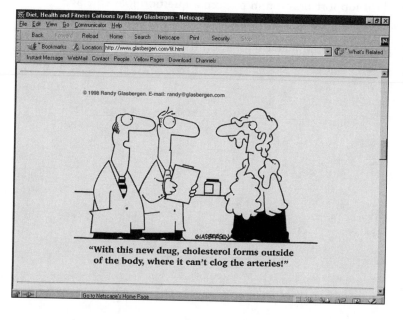

Figure 1.3

Randy Glasbergen spoofs health, fitness, and diet in his cartoons.

Medical Slips

`http://home3.swipnet.se/~w-37418/medslip.html`

"Bleeding started in the rectal area and continued all the way to Los Angeles." You'll laugh aloud at this collection of language slips from medical interview records written by various paramedics, emergency room receptionists, and the occasional doctor or two, all from major American hospitals.

Canonical List of Medical Humor (Funny Bone)

`http://www-personal.usyd.edu.au/~atan/jokes/canonical_medical.html`

500 medical jokes reside at this site, categorized by dentists, doctors, gynecologists, morticians, nurses, obstetricians, pharmacists, proctologists, psychiatrists, sex therapists, surgeons, and medicine. Some are the old jokes you have heard since childhood; others are irreverent, for adults only, and not for the easily offended!

The Least You Need to Know

➤ Do not use online medical information as a substitute for seeking medical help.

➤ Be discriminating in your choice of Web sites for medical information.

➤ You can get personal answers to your medical questions from a physician online, but don't go to the Internet for diagnosis or treatment.

➤ Finding a friend for support or a forum to pose a question is as easy as a mouse click when using mailing lists, newsgroups, bulletin boards, and chat.

➤ Take a break by reading some medical jokes on the Web.

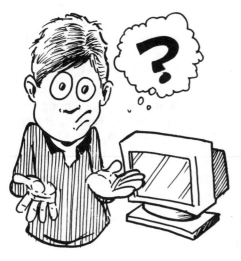

Chapter 2

Whom Can You Trust? Identifying Quality Information

In This Chapter

➤ Reading medical journals online

➤ Learning about Medscape and MEDLINE

➤ Using consumer health information from the government

This book is full of recommended medical sites that are trustworthy, interesting, welcoming, and easy to understand. But a book about online medical resources would be incomplete if it didn't also point you to the sources of medical information that your doctor reads: the medical journals and libraries of databases.

These sites are the most trustworthy—no one interprets the research for you, or decides what you learn and what you won't learn. It's all there. But I'd be lying if I told you that reading the research is easy—it's not. These sites aren't for casual skimming—use them if you know what you want to find, and when you want the most current and accurate information possible.

If trying to read information from these resources reminds you of your worst college nightmare—an exam on material you don't understand and in language that only vaguely resembles English—don't panic. This chapter also shows you some consumer-oriented sites that put medical research findings into reader-friendly articles for you.

Medical Journals: Read What Your Doctor Reads

All medical journals are not created equal. 16,000 peer-reviewed journals exist. Peer review means that experts in that topic analyze the studies carefully and decide whether they are worthy of publication.

Some medical journals are very selective; others aren't. At one extreme are the most respected journals, such as the *New England Journal of Medicine* (NEJM) and the *Journal of the American Medical Association* (JAMA). Articles are submitted by researchers with impressive credentials and academic skills. Lesser mortals don't even try to submit an article to these top guns. Even so, only one in 10 of these articles get accepted for publication. Others are sent back to the drawing board.

At the other extreme is the journal that accepts just about anything, like a hungry dog grateful for any morsel. If your source is a journal you've never heard of, don't figure that it's necessarily your ignorance—check it out with someone who knows medical journals, such as your doctor.

Don't Get Suckered

Be wary of sites that cite a journal that sounds almost—but not quite—like a well-known, respected journal. This could be a fictitious title created to confuse you. Example: *New England Medical Journal* is fake; *New England Journal of Medicine* is real. *Journal of the American Medical Society* is fake; *Journal of the American Medical Association* is real.

How to Find Medical Journals

The following sites help you find medical journals and other related resources on the Web.

MD Consult

`http://www.mdconsult.com`

Designed for medical professionals, this is a virtual library of medical textbooks and journals. You can search more than 35 leading medical books simultaneously, find full-text journal articles from 45 journals online, read about the latest developments in medicine, search for drugs, and read your choice of 2,600 patient handouts. **What Patients Are Reading** gives medical information about topics in the media, including synopses of *ER* episodes!

Medical and Scientific Journal Web Sites

`http://www.medlib.iupui.edu/techserv/ejournals.html`

Find out which medical and scientific journals have Web sites, and which of those offer full-text articles online. This site is from the medical library at the Indiana University School of Medicine.

Medical Journals Online

Some medical journals post their articles online. Others post the table of contents and abstracts (short summaries of the studies), but not the whole text of articles. Others charge a per-article fee, and it's usually well worth the small expense to learn about a study that is exactly on target.

Two of the most prestigious medical journals offer partial online access for nonsubscribers.

Journal of the American Medical Association

`http://www.jama.com`

You used to be able to read only abstracts online, but at the time of this writing, full-text articles of current and past issues are available to you online even if you're not a subscriber. Starting in April 2000, however, JAMA returns to partial access for non-subscribers. You'll still be able to read the table of contents and abstracts.

The New England Journal of Medicine

`http://www.nejm.org`

Read abstracts, tables of contents, correspondence, editorials, and book reviews for free each week. You can buy full-text individual articles, or, if you're a subscriber, you can read it all online (see Figure 2.1).

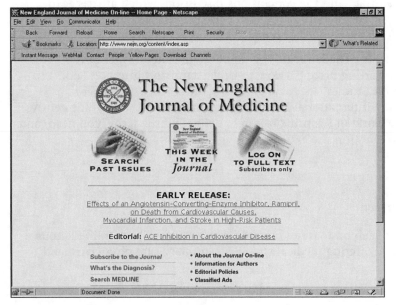

Figure 2.1

The New England Journal of Medicine Web site permits non-subscribers to read parts of each issue.

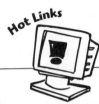

Your Own Medical Librarian

If you want a quick course in how to find and read medical journals or use MED-LINE, and you wish you had your own medical librarian, you do. Her name is Rochelle Perrine Schmalz, MSL (Masters Library Science), and she works for you at Dean Edell's HealthCentral. You can find a list of her columns at http://www.healthcentral.com. Click **columnists**, and then on the title of Ms. Schmalz's latest article, and from there, scroll down to the complete list of all her articles.

How to Understand Medical Journals

Medical journals are a challenge to read and even more of a challenge to understand. They are written for health professionals, not the general public, in scientific language that is intimidating—sometimes even incomprehensible—if you're unaccustomed to reading this kind of material.

Don't panic. Let the abstract and the conclusions/discussion, which are easier to understand, get you started. Take these to your physician, and ask for help understanding how the information you found relates to your medical care.

If you're ready to tackle the challenge of how to be an educated reader of the research, an excellent starting place is "How to Understand and Interpret Food and Health-Related Scientific Studies" (http://ificinfo.health.org/brochure/ificrevu.htm) from the International Food Information Council. This guide gently introduces you to the world of scientific research, defines all the terms you need, and even tells you how to question the experts.

Medscape

http://www.medscape.com

How does your doctor keep up to date? One way is Medscape, "The Online Resource for Better Patient Care," offering medical specialists, primary care physicians, and other health professionals "the Web's most robust and integrated multi-specialty medical information and education tool."

The continually updated, peer-reviewed content comes from tens of thousands of medical journal articles, medical meeting summaries, and more. You, as well as your physician, can use Medscape to learn the latest developments in 12 different specialties. Realize that the content is written for health professionals, not patients, so you might need your physician's help to understand the lingo.

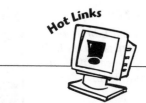

Hot Links

A Medscape User's Guide

`http://cardiology.medscape.`
`com/4691.rhtml`

Read this welcoming article from *Information Today* before doing a Medscape search—it makes the process easier.

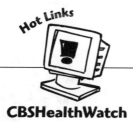

Hot Links

CBSHealthWatch

`http://healthwatch.medscape.com/`

Medscape's new consumer health site offers three tiers of accurate, up-to-date medical information: Basic-level articles and news (available without registration), Advanced, and What My Doctor Reads (both available with free registration).

MEDLINE

`http://igm.nlm.nih.gov`

MEDLINE is the online database from the National Library of Medicine (see Figure 2.2) that gives you access to the world's medical literature. MEDLINE contains more than 10 million references to journal articles from 4,300 journals in about 30 languages. 7,300 references are added weekly—almost 400,000 a year. You might have to pay for full-text articles, but the summaries are free.

If reading the medical literature is too daunting, click **MEDLINEplus** for consumer health information (or type `http://www.nlm.nih.gov/medlineplus/` directly) from the same source.

Figure 2.2

The National Library of Medicine offers access to the world's medical literature through MEDLINE.

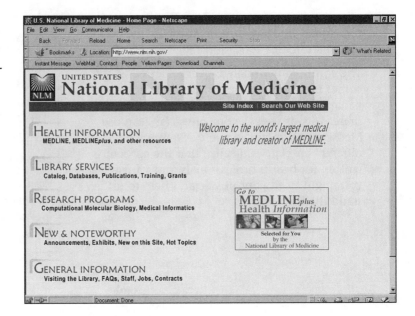

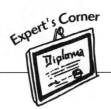

Expert's Corner

"For actual medical information, I always go to the source, the National Library of Medicine's online site: MEDLINE (`http://igm.nlm.nih.gov`). MEDLINE is easy to search by author, title words of the article, or subject. You can get title, author, and abstracts of almost any medical journal article. You might need a medical dictionary, but you can get the gist. You also get the first author's affiliation, so you can contact him/her. This is especially useful if you have a rare illness and are looking for an expert. I prefer to go to the source, review the research, and make up my own mind, rather than read second- or third-hand interpretation on some other site. And this is not as difficult as it might seem. Anyone can do it. Check it out."

—Michael Castleman, San Francisco–based medical journalist, author of 10 books and contributor to several health Web sites.

Consumer Education Medical Sites

Some excellent medical sites are developed with the sole purpose of educating consumers and are funded by our tax dollars at work. Others are related to hospitals, medical associations, and universities.

Still others are commercial sites that have a mission to present accurate information to the public. These commercial sites make money by selling ads to companies that are hungry to reach consumers who are interested in health. The reliable commercial sites are careful to keep advertising and medical content separate.

The "Medical Super Sites" described in Chapter 4, "How to Evaluate a Medical Site," and the sites recommended throughout the book represent an elite sampling of the best of all of these categories. They provide trustworthy, constantly updated, medical content. Visit them often!

Government Consumer Sites

The United States Government has regulatory agencies that attempt to protect our health and our wallets. Painfully understaffed and underfunded, these agencies realize that they can only protect us if they teach us to protect ourselves. They issue both print publications and online guides that are clear, comprehensive, and easy to understand. (Some are even fun to read!) The following are some online government resources.

FDA Consumer

`http://www.fda.gov/fdac/`

FDA Consumer, the official magazine of the U.S. Food and Drug Administration, is available as a print magazine for $12 a year or free online. This magazine is chockfull of excellent consumer information.

Don't miss **How to Spot Health Fraud** (`http://www.fda.gov/fdac/features/1999/699_fraud.html`) in the November/December 1999 issue. This article exposes fraudulent health claims using examples from three real products: emu oil ("extremely beneficial" in the treatment of rheumatism, arthritis, infections, prostate problems, ulcers, cancer, heart trouble, diabetes, and gangrene, and "eliminates skin cancer in days!"), an over-the-counter transdermal weight-loss patch ("[lose] 4 pounds each week"), and an unapproved weight-loss product marketed as a natural alternative to a hazardous prescription drug combination (see Figure 2.3).

Figure 2.3

FDA Consumer *points out fraudulent health claims from a weight-loss product.*

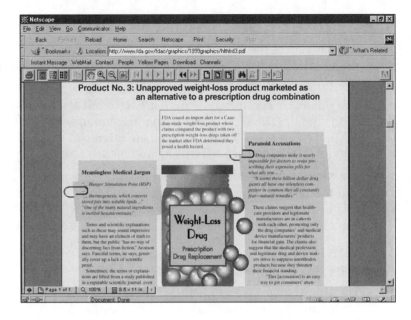

By the way, in case you're confused about the difference between the FDA (Food and Drug Administration) and the FTC (Federal Trade Commission), here it is from the horse's mouth: "FDA shares federal oversight of health fraud products with the Federal Trade Commission. FDA regulates safety, manufacturing and product labeling, including claims in labeling, such as package inserts and accompanying literature. FTC regulates advertising of these products."

Neither agency has the staff or the funding to keep up with Internet health fraud, so don't assume that if the government hasn't closed it down, a product is safe and effective. It's up to you to be your own watchdog.

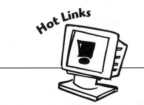

Hot Links

Government Publications

http://www.nlm.nih.gov/medlineplus/publicationsnews.html

This jump site from MEDLINEplus links to agencies that offer government-sponsored medical publications online. Don't skip this site because you think government health publications probably read like IRS tax instructions—they don't. The health publications are lively, helpful, and clear. (The IRS should borrow their writers.)

The Agency for Healthcare Research and Quality

http://www.ahcpr.gov/consumer/

The Agency for Healthcare Research and Quality (AHRQ), formerly the Agency for Health Care Policy and Research, is part of the U.S. Department of Health and Human Services. AHRQ supports research "designed to improve the quality of health care, reduce its cost, and broaden access to essential services." This site lists more than 30 excellent and comprehensive health guides available online on subjects as diverse as choosing a health plan, quitting smoking, controlling pain after surgery, recovering after a stroke, and several guides to specific diseases.

The Least You Need to Know

➤ You can get the most current medical information from the medical journals.

➤ MEDLINE and Medscape give you access to the same information your doctor reads.

➤ The government provides excellent online health guides.

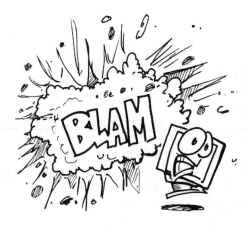

Chapter 3

Medical Minefield: Watching Where You Step

In This Chapter

➤ Understanding that misinformation masquerades as medical information

➤ Recognizing the signs of a quack site

➤ Spotting and resisting a sales pitch

➤ Protecting your privacy online

It's easy to spot a scam site when bold print in garish colors proclaims the merits of an expensive, unfamiliar product amidst misspellings, grammatical errors, and the vocabulary of a fifth grader.

It's not so easy to spot misinformation when it is presented by a self-proclaimed physician, or a patient who claims to have been cured of a disease, or a nicely crafted medical or alternative-health site. You know you can't believe everything you read, but you don't know how to tell which sites are minefields and which are minefields!

This chapter walks you safely over the minefields and teaches you to spot the danger signals.

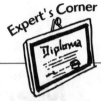

Caveat Surfer

"There's more bad information than good information out there. Miracles and 'breakthroughs' are not announced on the Internet. That simple, all-natural supplement to cure complex chronic illness does not exist. Double, no, *triple* check any advice with someone you trust and know to be knowledgeable. Do not do anything or take any advice from the Web that you do not check with your doctor first."

—Dean Edell, M.D., author of *Eat, Drink & Be Merry* (Harper Collins, 1999), http://www.healthcentral.com

What's the Problem?

The Web is a minefield because you can get misinformed, even dangerous, advice that affects your health as well as your wallet. Fraudulent medical sites can wear many faces. The following are a few examples:

➤ Slick Web sites that seem to be giving legitimate medical advice, but are actually trying to sell you a product.

➤ Emotional appeals that tell you what you want to hear and are hard to resist.

➤ Personal sites from people with your disease who claim to have been cured. These people might genuinely believe the therapy to be effective, even if it isn't.

➤ Credible medical content mixed with inaccurate, unproven, or outdated information.

➤ Convincing, seemingly reasonable advice from a medical professional who has a political agenda, a book or other product to sell, an axe to grind, or an earnest belief that only he or she has the truth.

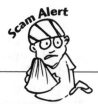

It's a Jungle

Only 47 percent of 160 randomly chosen health Web sites were produced by established health and consumer-education organizations, according to a study by Interactive Solutions. The rest were operated by consumers, sellers, manufacturers, and unidentified sources. Consumers produced one out of four health sites in 1998. But how do you know that whatever is being touted actually cured one person's cancer or caused another to drop 60 pounds, or if it did, that it will work for you? You don't. If a certain product or treatment intrigues you, substantiate the evidence—don't take one person's word for anything.

Who's Protecting You?

You are. The Internet is too huge and global to be regulated. The real answer is to educate yourself and remain vigilant so the scammers don't get a toehold and you don't get fooled by misinformation. Fortunately, some consumer-protection watchdog groups and government agencies are helping in two ways: alerting fraudulent sites to clean up their act or go away, and educating the public.

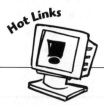

Internet "Carpetbaggers": What Are They Selling? Who's Watching?

http://www.acsh.org/publications/priorities/0903/internet.html

"The amount of health-related information, misinformation, and disinformation available on the Net is staggering." Learn why it is difficult or impossible to regulate health information on the Internet from this article by epidemiologist Ken Legins, M.P.H., from the American Council on Science and Health (ACSH).

Operation Cure.All

The Federal Trade Commission launched "Operation Cure.All" (http://www.ftc.gov/opa/1999/9906/opcureall.htm) in June 1999, a campaign aimed at curbing fraudulent health claims on the Internet. Operation Cure.All uses the Internet "both as a law enforcement tool to stop bogus claims for products and treatments touted as cures for various diseases and as a communication tool to provide consumers with good-quality health information," says the FTC.

The FTC got a running start by warning operators of 800 different Web sites and charging four companies with making deceptive and unsubstantiated health claims for "miracle cures" for serious illnesses. One advertised a beef-tallow arthritis cure, another shark cartilage capsules to cure cancer and AIDS/HIV, and two were magnetic therapy devices advertised to treat cancer, high blood pressure, and a wide variety of other ailments.

Can Operation Cure.All stop online health fraud? No, but it helps. As consumers become more knowledgeable, they're taken in less frequently. But we suspect that the companies will also get more knowledgeable at appealing to your emotions and hopes without breaking the letter of the law. Stay vigilant!

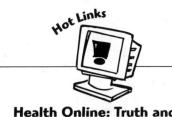

Health Online: Truth and Virtual Lies

http://www.msnbc.com/news/161811.asp

Charlene Laino of MSNBC presents experts' tips for distinguishing medical fact from fiction to help you figure out if the health information you find online is accurate.

Quackwatch

Quackwatch (http://www.quackwatch.com), "Your Guide to Health Fraud, Quackery, and Intelligent Decisions," is an enormous, amazing Web site operated by Stephen Barrett, M.D. (see Figure 3.1). Dr. Barrett is on a crusade to "combat health-related frauds, myths, fads, and fallacies," especially on the Internet. He posts hundreds of articles aimed at educating you and protecting you from fraud. Read listings in categories such as Questionable Products, Services, and Theories; Questionable Advertisements (Illustrated); Unrecommended Sources of Health Advice; and Consumer Strategies.

If you already are a regular or irregular visitor to Quackwatch and are overwhelmed by the amount of information (650 pages and counting), http://www.quackwatch.com/00AboutQuackwatch/new.html lists the newest additions and updated articles.

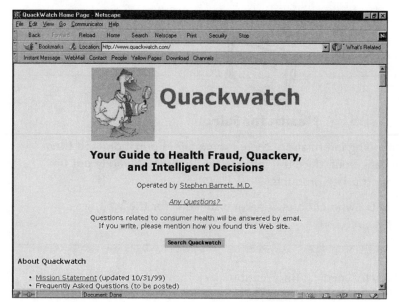

Figure 3.1

Quackwatch warns you about fraudulent sites and products.

If It Quacks Like a Quack... Recognizing the Red Flags

Clever marketers use the Web to make science and snake oil appear equally true. Consumers who are desperate for answers to their medical problems can often be easily swayed by fraudulent claims or earnest, but worthless, opinions. Protect yourself by learning about the quackery and fraud that is abundant online. Watch for the following signs that you're not reading credible medical information.

Send Money!

The Web is full of misinformation and products that claim to perform miracles on your body. Restore sexual potency to teenage vigor! Turn a bald pate into a full head of curly hair! Cure cancer with the secret your doctor doesn't want you to know! Each year, consumers waste billions of dollars on unproven, fraudulently marketed, and sometimes unsafe, health and fitness products.

We all hope that suddenly there will be a miracle cure, a fountain of youth, or a magic bullet to remedy all of our health concerns. But the truth is there is no magic cure for incurable diseases, and there is no treatment that cures a variety of unrelated diseases (that's not the way things work), so don't waste your cash.

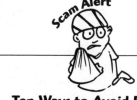

Ten Ways to Avoid Being Quacked

http://www.quackwatch.com/
01QuackeryRelatedTopics/
avoid.html

This article, written by Stephen Barrett, M.D., gives you 10 strategies for recognizing a quack Web site.

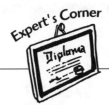

Health for Sale

"There's some outstanding information, there's some fair information, and then there's some really dangerous, deceitful information that's deliberately put up there to market inappropriate products."

—John H. Renner, M.D., who chooses "stars and stinkers" for the Web site `http://www.healthscout.com/`.

When you surf the Web for medical information, keep in mind one basic fact: Companies are out there to make money. They don't know you, and most don't care about your plight. They just want your money. With e-commerce becoming more and more common, a company selling a product doesn't have to see you face-to-face or even speak to you on the phone. Con artists happily take your money right over the Internet in a completely anonymous rip-off.

"But there's a money-back guarantee!" you insist. Guess what? A scam artist is in the business of selling you with soothing, hopeful words. Who do you think enforces that money-back guarantee? They might not even be in business anymore after taking a significant amount of money from unsuspecting customers. Besides, most people who realize they were bilked are too embarrassed to try to get their money back.

Trash That Email!

Never buy a product you learn about from an unsolicited email. No cancer discovery or impotence cure will ever be announced first in a mass emailing. Scam, scam, scam.

The Truth No One Wants You to Know!!!

This is such bunk that it's a wonder that people fall for it. These sites claim that the "truth" is being hidden by the "medical establishment," a government conspiracy, or some other group. What is this "truth"? A "cure" for cancer, AIDS, arthritis, or all of these. Uh uh. No truth to it.

These sites sometimes claim that the American Medical Association or the "medical establishment" (whatever that is) doesn't want you to know that the cure for cancer (for example) exists, because doctors would stop making money. Please! Your doctor does not have an investment in keeping patients sick. Besides, if your oncologist knew of a treatment that honestly cured cancer, don't you think he or she would be offering it? You couldn't keep patients away.

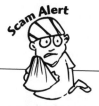

Email Health Hoaxes

Does anyone understand what kind of people get their kicks by starting email health scares? They've come up with some doozies. Here's the truth about a few common ones:

➤ Waterproof sunscreen will not make your children go blind.

➤ Antiperspirants do not cause breast cancer.

➤ Aspartame does not cause multiple sclerosis or lupus.

➤ HIV-infected needles are not being found in telephone coin returns or movie theaters.

➤ Tampons do not contain asbestos.

➤ Shampoo does not cause cancer.

Before you swallow a medical scare story that you read on the Internet—especially when it comes to you via email from a worried friend who got it from a worried friend who got it from...you get the idea—check out the health hoaxes and urban rumors that are making the rounds and freaking people. If you want to check the authenticity of these or any other hair-raising health warnings you might read on the Internet, Dr. Dean Edell has a bunch of reports at http://www.healthcentral.com. Click **Hot Topics**, and then **Internet Hoax Watch**.

If you get an email that warns you about some awful health consequence of an innocuous product or ordinary behavior, just delete it, even if it comes from your high-school sweetheart. And please, when it implores you to send it to your entire mailing list (and it will), don't! Especially when it has a lot of exclamation points!!!!!!

Scientific Breakthrough!

Scientific breakthroughs happen in movies, not real life. Medical progress takes time. Sudden discoveries that have immediate medical applications are rare indeed.

This process involves a long, tedious research process that is carefully documented. A study is then submitted to a respected medical journal, and carefully examined by medical professionals (peer reviewed). A few make it past the peer-review process into publication.

Even when research points to a promising treatment, the findings need to be replicated. That means it still has to be studied again and again, to see if those results can be duplicated, and what unexpected results might emerge.

There's no "breakthrough" possible here. Run from sites that advertise a treatment or cure that is so new that even your doctor hasn't heard about it—it just doesn't work that way.

Besides, if there really was a breakthrough cure for cancer or AIDS, would it be announced in a commercial Web site first? Of course not! You'd see all the networks and newspapers racing to announce it first.

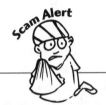

Don't Answer Spam

If you get spam and it gives a "respond-to" address to get off the mailing list, don't respond! They're just trying to find out which of the email addresses they bought (or found randomly) are "live." If you respond, your email address gets used and sold over and over again. Most ISPs and online services have an email address for reporting spam. Forward unwanted and annoying spam to that address, and then delete it.

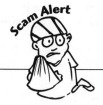

Beware of Buzzwords

These buzzwords are hot buttons that set off dreams and emotions, not your reason. They are red flags that warn you to evaluate the information with your head, not your hopes:

➤ Ancient

➤ Best

➤ Breakthrough

➤ Cure

➤ Magic

➤ Miracle

➤ Natural

➤ No side effects

➤ Only

➤ Secret

If It Sounds Too Good to Be True, It Probably Is

This is your new mantra as you surf the Web for quality health and fitness information. Ask yourself this question: If there really was a medical breakthrough, secret ingredient, or ancient remedy, would it hide in a Web site advertisement? If there really was a product that cured every ailment from arthritis to zits, would it be announced by email spam?

Of course not. These scientists would be publishing in the most prestigious medical journals and hoping for the Nobel prize!

You read about the many people who've had success on a certain program or with a certain product. Forget it. Anyone can say anything.

Even if they're telling the truth—or think they are—they might have gotten better while using the potion or herb or device, but do you know the whole story? What else were these people doing while they drank the ancient elixir or wore the magic bracelet? Maybe they were also on other medications. Maybe their disease went into spontaneous remission. Maybe they are the product seller's in-laws. Maybe they don't even exist. Never pin your hopes for disease cure on a product that sounds too good to be true, because it usually is.

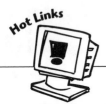

Hot Links

Why Bogus Therapies Often Seem to Work

```
http://www.quackwatch.com/
01QuackeryRelatedTopics/
altbelief.html
```

This article by biopsychologist Barry L. Beyerstein, Ph.D., describes seven reasons why people might get better and think an ineffective therapy works, even when it doesn't.

Buy Me: Products for Sale

If a site is selling products, be aware of potential bias in the type and slant of information you get. Does the content promote the products? Or is the content carefully kept separate and based on science rather than profit?

The medical information you read on a site that accepts advertising is not necessarily suspect. Many of the "Medical Super Sites" in this book accept advertising to survive, because other funding sources don't support them. Someone has to pay for the site, and thank goodness, it's not the viewer! Their medical information can be credible, as long as they clearly separate advertising and editorial content. Reputable sites that do accept advertising issue a policy statement about advertising not influencing editorial content.

But sniff hard for any signs that a site's medical information is slanted toward product promotion, and adjust your trust meter accordingly.

The extreme "Buy Me!" sites are the snake-oil schemes (not that they make it easy by labeling them as such). If a so-called medical article promotes one weird product, or is using high-powered sales tactics to get you to buy NOW!!!!, cross this site off your list. Hide your credit card—ESPECIALLY IF IT USES CAPITAL LETTERS AND EXCLAMATION POINTS!!!!!!!

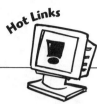

Hot Links

Privacy in Cyberspace: Rules of the Road for the Information Superhighway

`http://www.privacyrights.org/FS/fs18-cyb.htm`

"There are virtually no online activities or services that guarantee an absolute right of privacy." Before you drive the information superhighway, learn the "privacy rules of the road" to make sure your online activity doesn't lead to significant privacy problems. This revealing fact sheet from Privacy Rights Clearinghouse also has links to other privacy sites.

Protecting Your Privacy Online

How private is your Web surfing? Not very. The sites you visit might be collecting information about which pages of the site you visit, which other Web sites you've browsed, sometimes even your email address. Your own service provider might be tracking this information. And all this is done without a whisper of informed consent.

When you surf the Web, a site you visit might drop data on your hard drive (these are called "cookies," and they don't have chocolate chips). When you return to the same site, the cookie data tells the site that you've been there before and retrieves whatever information might be stored about you.

This isn't always bad. If you're storing your medical record on a site, you want it to be there when you return, and you don't want to jump through hoops to retrieve it. If you've ordered from an online bookstore before and you want to order again, or you've subscribed to a site, you want to zip your way through without hassles. Cookies mean you never have to enter the same information over and over again. It's really quite handy—*if* (and only if) it's your choice!

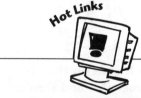

Hot Links

Rules and Tools for Protecting Personal Privacy Online

`http://www.privacyalliance.com/resources/rulesntools.shtml`

You can take steps to prevent your personal information from being gathered when you surf, shop, and chat online. This site spells out what to do—and what *not* to do.

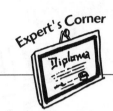

Expert's Corner

Protect Your Privacy

"Few things are more personal and private than health information. It's important that consumers are aware of the need to use caution when posting personal information to the Web, and know what to look for when choosing a health site. Currently, there is no standardization of privacy policies for health sites. The best sites are up-front with their privacy policies and subscribe to organizations that provide guidelines for privacy protection, such as the TRUSTe Privacy Program. Not all health sites on the Internet take measures to ensure the privacy of its users."

—Raj Lakhanpal, M.D., founder and president of healthAtoZ.com (www.healthAtoZ.com)

But do you really want a site you've visited to collect data on your online "browsing patterns" to sell to marketers? This is a common practice.

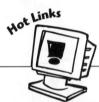

Hot Links

Playing It Safe on the Web: Consumer Dos and Don'ts

http://www.truste.org/users/users_primer.html

Read TRUSTe's collection of "commonsense rules and take-charge tips for safeguarding your privacy online" as they relate to a number of your concerns, including children, cookies, and chat rooms.

You can protect yourself somewhat by reading a site's privacy policy statements and learning which sites protect your privacy and don't sell your information to marketers. The Federal Trade Commission is encouraging commercial Web sites to reveal their privacy or information-collecting policies clearly and openly. Many do this; many do not.

A good sign is a posted privacy "seal of approval," such as TRUSTe (http://www.truste.org), on the home page. The TRUSTe logo means that the site agrees to post its privacy policies and submit to oversight of its privacy practices (see Figure 3.2). Another reputable privacy seal is from BBB: the Council of Better Business Bureaus (http://www.bbbonline.org).

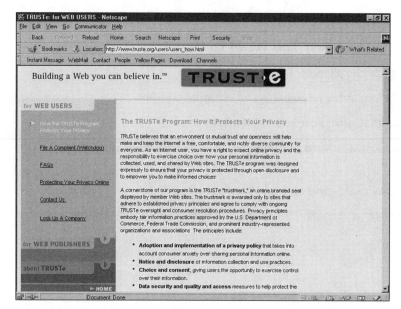

Figure 3.2
TRUSTe helps protect consumer privacy.

Of course, if you're browsing from site to site, exploring or collecting information, you can't always stick to sites that won't sell you out. Inform yourself as much as possible, and don't post anything private. Realize that any messages you post to a public newsgroup or message board can be viewed, copied, stored, and even forwarded to others, by anyone.

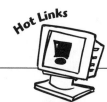

Smart Choices: Fraud and Complaints—How to Recognize a Quack or Scam

http://www.healthfinder.gov/smartchoices/fraud/quack.htm

Do you wish this chapter was longer because you want to learn more about online health fraud? Check out this site from HealthFinder, which links to articles about online and offline health frauds and the Web pages of organizations that protect you from them.

The Least You Need to Know

➤ Learn to recognize the signs of a quack Web site.

➤ Make sure a site separates advertising and editorial content.

➤ Be wary of sites that want you to send money.

➤ Be careful not to post private information on the Internet—it isn't really private.

➤ Look for a privacy policy and seal on the sites you visit.

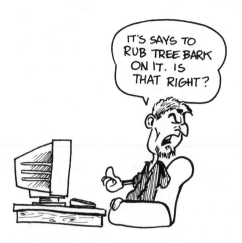

Chapter 4

How to Evaluate a Medical Site

In This Chapter

➤ Tips for figuring out whether the medical information you find online is sound

➤ How to evaluate medical Web sites using the PILOT Method

➤ Understanding the HONcode

➤ Exploring the Web with a selection of Medical Super Sites

There's good news and bad news about finding medical information online. The good news is that there is an almost unlimited amount of information. The bad news is that there is an almost unlimited amount of information!

You can get an unfamiliar medical diagnosis one day, and before your next appointment (or by the next day, depending on your determination and stamina), you might know more about your condition than most health professionals, including your own doctor. You can read the same research studies that your doctor does (or would, if he or she had time), search medical libraries, and "talk" to other patients with that the same condition.

But be cautious—because you don't have the medical background to evaluate the information you find, you might also be swayed by unproven treatments, misinformed by out-of-date information, or even bilked by conwebs (Shannon Entin and I invented that word for *The Complete Idiot's Guide to Online Health and Fitness*: Web sites run by con artists).

This chapter teaches you how to evaluate medical Web sites with the easy, step-by-step PILOT method introduced in *The Complete Idiot's Guide to Online Health and Fitness*.

Then you get a gift worth the price of the book: an annotated list of "Medical Super Sites" that are trustworthy, full of information, and well worth many visits.

Evaluating Web Site Content

Okay, you carefully read Chapter 3, "Medical Minefield: Watching Where You Step," and you feel confident that you won't fall for scummy sites. But what about sites that *seem* reputable? How can you tell if they really are?

The Web makes it simple for just about anyone—physicians, patients, researchers, vendors, kooks, ex-cons, your 13-year-old cousin, or that weird neighbor who invents things that go boom in his basement—to disseminate useful or useless information. It's often difficult to distinguish between reliable content and entertainment or advertising. Quick and easy access to virtually boundless medical information has its benefits, but it also has serious drawbacks. Some advice can be downright harmful.

How reliable is the information you find on the Internet? That depends. It can be completely reliable and exceedingly useful, but you need to learn how to evaluate the Web site that interests you.

Trust Your Gut

If a site is poorly organized and unattractive, that might be a major clue that the creator of the site is not professional enough to design a nice-looking, user-friendly Web page. Likewise, if the site is riddled with numerous colors, blinking words, exclamation points, or flashing graphics to the point that it's difficult to discern the content, those are sometimes indicators of quack sites. These elements don't prove that the site was put up by a bunch of lowlifes snickering in their basement or a "loony toon" who can't get anyone else to listen, but do you really want to trust this person with your health decisions? User experience—the organization, flow, and overall "feel" of the site—should be a factor in your evaluation.

The PILOT Method

To help you PILOT your way through the friendly skies of World Wide Web health information, Shannon Entin and I developed a method for evaluating Web site content for *The Complete Idiot's Guide to Online Health and Fitness*. It's equally applicable here.

This systematic approach helps you quickly weed out the truly useless information and zero in on content you can trust:

P **Purpose**

I **Information**

L **Links**

O **Originator**

T **Timeliness**

Purpose

You're looking for sites that have one major purpose: to educate the public. Ideally, the purpose or mission is clearly stated. If not, it should be easy to interpret from the type of information presented.

If the site has a mission statement, read it. (It might be called "Mission," "Who Are We?," "About Us," or something similar.) If not, read the home page and analyze the site's purpose. Does it inform, persuade, sell, outrage, or entertain? Ask yourself these questions:

➤ Does the site aim to educate people with articles and/or research that inform fairly?

➤ Is the site trying to sell you something? Be especially wary if this site is the only source for this product.

➤ Is it trying to convince you that one opinion is better than another?

➤ Is the site a personal page, designed as an outlet for someone's personal medical regimen or views?

➤ What can you tell about the site's target audience?

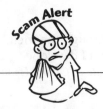

Keep Your Money

Does the site charge a fee for information about a product or plan? Keep your wallet firmly planted in your purse or back pocket. Certainly, some reputable sites do charge a fee to cover their expenses if they offer access to large volumes of medical information, or a subscription fee for their journal or organization. But a site that wants to charge you for the greatest arthritis discovery, or the cancer cure that the medical establishment doesn't want you to know, or a sexual potency breakthrough? Hogwash.

Information

Truly useful Web sites offer valuable information. That means more than advertising or splashy graphics. Be aware that advertising might be cleverly disguised as an article or "scientific research."

Few consumers have the background to evaluate the scientific validity of medical information, but there's still a lot you can do to increase the chances that the information you're reading is helpful and accurate. Here are some questions you should ponder:

➤ Is the content fact, supported by documented research, credible sources, or authoritative references? Or are undocumented case histories used as "proof" to substantiate claims?

➤ Is this science or fluff? What research is cited? Has the research been published in a peer-reviewed journal? Are the "facts" backed by sources and references, and not simply by anecdote?

➤ Does a scientific or medical advisory board oversee the medical content?

➤ Is the content propaganda, designed to persuade you and appeal to your emotions? If so, resist.

➤ Is this fact or opinion? If it's opinion, who or what is the source, and is this opinion supported by other credible sources? Are opposing sides presented?

➤ If the site is selling or advertising a product, plan, or service, how much is the content biased toward what's being sold? Does the site have a policy statement about the relationship between its advertising and its editorial content?

➤ Has the site won any awards? If so, from whom? What are the criteria for winning the award?

➤ Does this site claim to be the "only" or "best" source of information about this topic? Reputable sites do not claim to be the sole resource and do not disrespect other credible sources of knowledge.

➤ Can you find the same information repeated on other sites, especially government-, hospital-, or association-sponsored sites? How does this finding fit with other existing research? If the information is unique to one site, be wary!

Links

The best sites want to inform you and are happy to recommend additional Web sites to further your knowledge in that topic or related topics.

A site that holds you captive rather than sharing you with other sites is suspect. The best medical sites link with other sites that they've reviewed and know to be credible. But be wary of those that don't discriminate and link to anything that glows (or to those that reciprocate, regardless of quality).

Look for the following link qualities:

➤ Are the selected links recommended, related, and reliable sites? Random sites that run the gamut from credible to incredible might be fun on a rainy afternoon, but are frustrating when you're looking for the best information swiftly.

➤ Look for sites that organize their links into helpful categories, or better yet, include a rating and/or review.

➤ Be sure the links are up to date—if you click on a few and they're "dead" (no longer operational), move on to another site.

➤ Be wary of sites that have an "add your own link" feature or a long list of banners, sometimes unrelated to the topic. These serve only to drive more traffic to the Web site—they don't further your education/research of your topic.

Originator

Before you take any advice found on the Internet, determine who is responsible for the information. Who owns this site? Who sponsors it? Who advertises on it? Is any reputable hospital, association, or consumer agency affiliated with it? Is all of this readily apparent on the Web site?

Best bets for sound medical information are consumer advocacy groups, health professional organizations, well-known hospitals, and government- and university-sponsored sites. Some exceptional commercial sites also exist—such as the "Medical Super Sites" listed at the end of this chapter.

Ask the following questions to learn more about the originator:

➤ Who is responsible for the information? Look for an individual's name or the name of an organization.

➤ If the originator is an organization, what does it stand for and whom does it represent?

➤ If the originator is a person, what are his or her credentials, occupation, and affiliation? Does the author have the experience and authority to provide this information?

➤ What credentials do the experts have who write or oversee the content? Are they doctors or medical researchers? Are several experts quoted? Or are the so-called experts just people who have used a product and earnestly want you to benefit as they claim they have?

➤ Is the originator affiliated with a specific product or program? Is the site financially tied to a commercial venture through sponsorship, advertising, or underwriting? (If so, there still might be great information on the site if it passes the rest of our test, but take "proof" that a certain product is the best with many grains of salt.)

➤ Can you contact the originator by email or other means? The most reputable organizations/site publishers disclose full addresses and phone numbers so they can be contacted.

➤ Is the site run by a physician or health guru who diagnoses, treats, or prescribes online? Be skeptical.

Timeliness

Medical knowledge changes so fast that the information on a medical site *must* be current. Research is changing treatment recommendations and medications so rapidly that it's imperative to keep up.

For example, a medical site with out-of-date information could list a drug as safe even though it has recently been found to cause dangerous side effects; or a site might tout a treatment as effective that is now considered worthless.

A benefit of the Internet is how quickly information can be updated. You can see the latest data at the same time your medical professional sees it. You can read a new recommendation before it hits the newspaper or the evening news.

A savvy Web site might post an in-depth report about a new treatment months before print magazines present it, and a year before a book comes out on the topic. A drug site can update patient information instantly when new research is published about side effects and therapeutic interactions.

Check the date of any article or study you read, and if the information is not based on new studies, be sure the site is updated frequently enough that if there were anything new, you'd read about it. Don't assume that just because you're at a medical training hospital site, for example, it must be up to date—a recent study found several that were not updated diligently.

Examine the medical sites you visit with the following questions in mind:

➤ Is the content current? Look for dates in bylines of articles, or look for current issues on publication Web sites.

➤ How often is the site updated? Ideally, a site with time-sensitive health information should be updated daily, weekly, or monthly. Look for a policy statement about how often the site is updated.

➤ If the information has not been updated recently, is this material that you can trust not to go out of date?

What's the HONcode?

HONcode, which stands for Health On the Net Code of Conduct, is an ethical code for medical and health Web sites. More and more reputable sites—2,500 so far—are choosing to adopt this international code of conduct. Sites that wish to subscribe to the HONcode must make an application. Those that are judged as conforming to the eight principles of the honor code may display the HONcode symbol.

The HONcode does not rate the quality or the content provided by a Web site. Its purpose is to "define a set of rules designed to make sure the reader always knows the source and the purpose of the data he's reading."

The HONcode includes the following eight principles, as spelled out at `http://www.hon.ch/HONcode/Conduct.html`:

1. Any medical/health advice provided and hosted on this site will only be given by medically/health-trained and -qualified professionals unless a clear statement is made that a piece of advice offered is from a non-medically/health-qualified individual/organization.

2. The information provided on this site is designed to support, not replace, the relationship that exists between a patient/site visitor and his/her existing physician.

3. Confidentiality of data relating to individual patients and visitors to a medical/health Web site, including their identities, is respected by this Web site. The Web site owners undertake to honor or exceed the legal requirements of medical/health information privacy that apply in the country and state where the Web site and mirror sites are located.

4. Where appropriate, information contained on this site will be supported by clear references to source data and, where possible, have specific HTML links to that data. The date when a clinical page was last modified will be clearly displayed (for example, at the bottom of the page).

5. Any claims relating to the benefits/performance of a specific treatment, commercial product, or service will be supported by appropriate, balanced evidence in the manner outlined above in Principle 4.

6. The designers of this Web site will seek to provide information in the clearest possible manner and provide contact addresses for visitors that seek further information or support. The Webmaster will display his/her email address clearly throughout the Web site.

7. Support for this Web site will be clearly identified, including the identities of commercial and non-commercial organizations that have contributed funding, services, or material for the site.

8. If advertising is a source of funding, it will be clearly stated. A brief description of the advertising policy adopted by the Web site owners will be displayed on the site. Advertising and other promotional material will be presented to viewers in a manner and context that facilitates differentiation between it and the original material created by the institution operating the site.

Medical Super Sites

When you surf for medical Web sites, stick to the most reputable. Now that you're armed with information on finding and evaluating medical and health sites, start your own research with the following content sites and jump sites.

Content Sites

The best medical content sites are chockfull of reputable, science-based, up-to-date information. The following sites represent what a consumer medical site ought to be: accurate, thorough, up to date, and easy to understand.

adam.com

```
http://www.adam.com
```

adam.com has thousands of pages of medical content, news, illustrations, discussions, and interactive tools. Much of the site is a medical encyclopedia, with short, simple entries on each condition. What makes adam.com stand out are the medical illustrations, especially the illustrations of 45 surgeries.

allHealth from iVillage

```
http://www.allhealth.com/
```

iVillage's health channel has a wealth of medical information presented in comprehensive conditions centers, articles, news, chats, advice from experts, message boards, tools, and a drug database. iVillage ("The Women's Network") gives content with a sense of community.

drkoop.com

http://drkoop.com

Medical information from a variety of credible providers, ratings of other sites, more than 130 chat support groups, and interactive tools—you find all of this at this huge site. Dr. C. Everett Koop, the former U.S. Surgeon General, is co-founder and Chairman of the Board.

HealthAnswers.com

http://healthanswers.com

A profusion of health information, HealthAnswers.com covers 4,000 chronic disease and health topics with news and feature articles, a medical reference library, a bilingual (Spanish/English) pharmaceutical database, photos, chats, message boards, and tools. Look up a disease, and read a detailed explanation with symptoms, treatments, prognosis, complications, plus related articles, news releases, and drug recalls.

HealthAtoZ

http://www.healthatoz.com

HealthAtoZ, "your family health site," was developed by health-care professionals to provide an abundance of health/medical information, links to reviewed health sites, interactive tools, news, message boards, and chats (see Figure 4.1). You can store your medical record here and get email reminders.

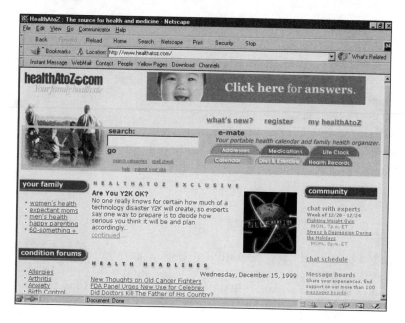

Figure 4.1

HealthAtoZ provides medical information for the whole family.

HealthCentral

`http://www.healthcentral.com`

This huge site has constantly updated, accurate information, with Dr. Dean Edell's spin on new medical studies, research reports, trends, and scams. "At HealthCentral I work to interpret, not just report, the latest medical news. You need opinion and interpretation, and my job is to give it to you," says "America's favorite doctor." The site also recaps all topics and questions and answers from his daily radio program.

InteliHealth

`http://www.intelihealth.com`

Read medical news and articles at this enormous, well-respected, award-winning, snazzy site from Johns Hopkins University and Health System and Aetna U.S. Healthcare. InteliHealth's "condition centers" are particularly valuable, with in-depth information on a variety of diseases and conditions (see Figure 4.2).

Figure 4.2

InteliHealth provides in-depth information on a variety of diseases and conditions.

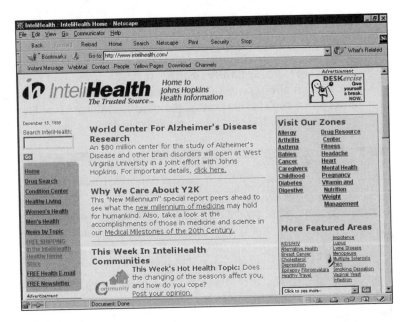

LaurusHealth

`http://www.laurushealth.com/`

LaurusHealth was founded by a national cooperative of 1,850 community-owned hospitals to provide consumer medical content. Read in-depth guides on more than 450 health conditions, and information about 2,400 prescription medications and 200 medical tests.

Mayo Clinic Health Oasis

http://www.mayohealth.org

"Reliable information for a healthier life," promises Mayo Clinic Health Oasis; and it delivers, offering medical news, quizzes, links, and a comprehensive selection of reference articles from 1,200 physicians and scientists (see Figure 4.3).

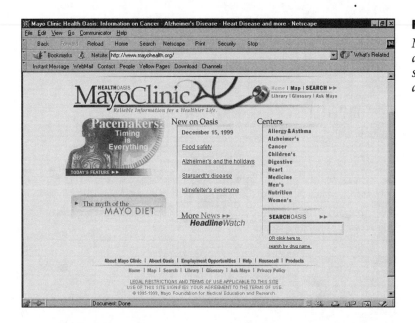

Figure 4.3

Mayo Clinic Health Oasis delivers a comprehensive selection of reference articles.

Mediconsult

http://www.mediconsult.com

Mediconsult's comprehensive condition centers offer in-depth and up-to-date patient information about many chronic medical conditions, as well as research, support, clinical trials, drug information, journal references, reviewed links, and more.

MEDLINE

http://igm.nlm.nih.gov

MEDLINE, from the world's largest biomedical library, the National Library of Medicine at the National Institutes of Health, gives you access to the world's medical literature. If that's too daunting, click **MEDLINEplus** for consumer health information from the same source, or go directly to http://www.nlm.nih.gov/medlineplus/.

OnHealth

http://www.onhealth.com

OnHealth presents thousands of pages of lively health information from Cleveland Clinic; Beth Israel Deaconess Medical Center; physicians who teach at Harvard, Columbia, and Stanford; and the publishers of the *New England Journal of Medicine* (see Figure 4.4).

Figure 4.4

OnHealth offers expert information in a readable style.

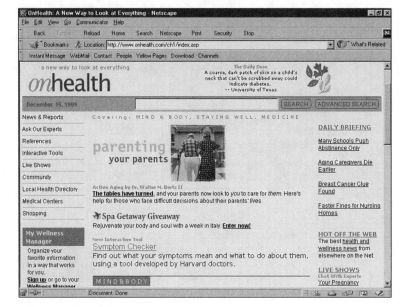

WebMDHealth

http://my.webmd.com

This site is a resource center for articles about every health/disease/health-care topic you can imagine (see Figure 4.5). WebMDHealth also offers live events, support, illustrations, and a variety of Health-O-Meters to track ovulation, delivery due date, target heart rate, health risk assessment, and more.

WellnessWeb

http://wellweb.com

WellnessWeb is a collaboration of patients, health-care professionals, and other caregivers "trying to put the HEART back in health care." Choose from a large selection of science-based medical information, plus some alternative content (clearly separated). Read late-breaking research, or join one of the WellnessWeb communities for chats.

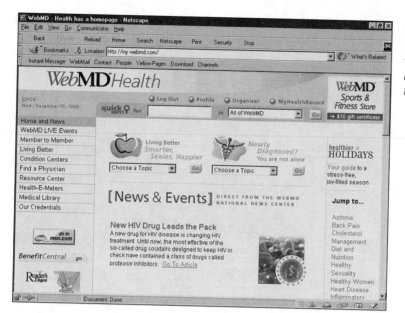

Figure 4.5
*WebMDHealth has a
wealth of information
about all areas of
medicine and health.*

Jump Sites

Jump sites provide categorized listings of links to other sites, rather than their own content. A jump site is most useful when the included sites are carefully screened by experts in the field. The following exemplary sites present only screened, valuable links.

Hardin Meta Directory of Internet Health Sources

`http://www.lib.uiowa.edu/hardin/md/index.html`

"We list the best sites that list the sites." This directory from the Hardin Library for the Health Sciences University of Iowa links to other well-maintained health jump sites that keep their links updated. This respected site has enough information to keep you clicking away all day.

Healthfinder

`http://www.healthfinder.gov`

This site is "a free gateway to reliable consumer health and human services information" developed by the U.S. Department of Health and Human Services. Healthfinder (see Figure 4.6) leads you to selected online publications, clearinghouses, databases, Web sites, support and self-help groups, government agencies, and not-for-profit organizations, all selected for their reliable information. 3,200 links in all! No advertising, no sales, no commercial links. This is a great starting place for information on any general health topic.

Figure 4.6

Healthfinder is a gateway to screened health sites.

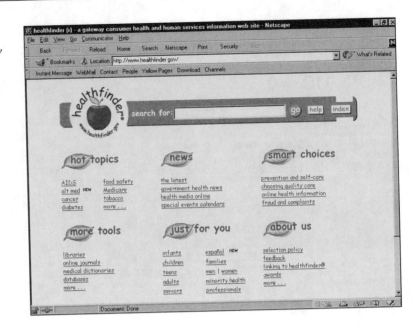

HealthWeb

`http://healthweb.org/`

HealthWeb provides annotated links to Web resources selected and evaluated by librarians and information professionals at academic medical centers in the Midwest. Click **subjects** to see a list of medical topics. This site serves health professionals as well as consumers, so after you've clicked a particular topic, click **patient information** if it's available.

New York Online Access to Health (NOAH)

`http://www.noah.cuny.edu`

NOAH is a team effort from the City University of New York, the Metropolitan New York Library Council, the New York Academy of Medicine, and the New York Public Library. It is primarily a jump site with many reviewed links for every health/medical topic imaginable, and it also has its own content. All information is available in both English and Spanish.

StayHealthy.com

`http://www.stayhealthy.com/`

StayHealthy has some health news and articles, but what makes this site outstanding is its useful links, annotated with ratings and reviews. Choose a disease, condition, or other health topics, and get a selection of screened links and book recommendations.

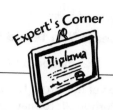

Finding Quality Health Information on the Internet: Tips for Health Consumers

The Internet Healthcare Coalition (www.ihealthcoalition.org) offers the following tips for evaluating the reliability of online health information and advice:

➤ Choosing an online health information resource is like choosing your doctor. You wouldn't go to just any doctor, and you might get opinions from several doctors. Therefore, you shouldn't rely on just any one Internet site for all your health needs. A good rule of thumb is to find a Web site that has a person, institution, or organization in which you already have confidence. If possible, you should seek information from several sources and not rely on a single source of information.

➤ Trust what you see or read on the Internet only if you can validate the source of the information. Authors and contributors should always be identified, along with their affiliations and financial interests, if any, in the content. Phone numbers, email addresses, or other contact information should also be provided.

➤ Question Web sites that credit themselves as the sole source of information on a topic, as well as sites that disrespect other sources of knowledge.

➤ Don't be fooled by a comprehensive list of links. Any Web site can link to another and this in no way implies endorsement from either site.

➤ Find out if the site is professionally managed and reviewed by an editorial board of experts to ensure that the material is both credible and reliable. Sources used to create the content should be clearly referenced and acknowledged.

➤ Medical knowledge is continually evolving. Make sure that all clinical content includes the date of publication or modification.

➤ Any and all sponsorship, advertising, underwriting, commercial funding arrangements, or potential conflicts should be clearly stated and separated from the editorial content. A good question to ask is: Does the author or authors have anything to gain from proposing one particular point of view over another?

➤ Avoid any online physician who proposes to diagnose or treat you without a proper physical examination and consultation regarding your medical history.

➤ Read the Web site's privacy statement and make certain that any personal medical or other information you supply will be kept absolutely confidential.

➤ Most importantly, use your common sense! Shop around, always get more than one opinion, be suspicious of miracle cures, and always read the fine print.

The Least You Need to Know

➤ Don't just accept medical information on the Web—evaluate its credibility.

➤ Weed out the medical jewel sites from the junk sites by using the PILOT method of evaluation: Purpose, Information, Links, Originator, and Timeliness.

➤ The HONcode seal indicates that the site subscribes to an international code of ethics.

➤ Start with the "Medical Super Sites" in this chapter to start your online exploration of a medical topic.

Part 2

You and Your Medical Care

Are you looking for health insurance? The right hospital for a particular procedure? A physician in a certain specialty? A source for diabetes supplies or disability aids?

The chapters in Part 2 help you brace up your own personal medical care with Internet resources that can help you make the best choices. You learn how to enlist the power of the Internet to learn about and choose health care, buy medical supplies, and make your physician your partner.

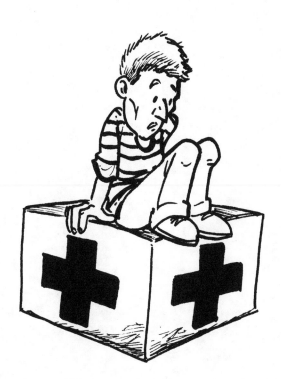

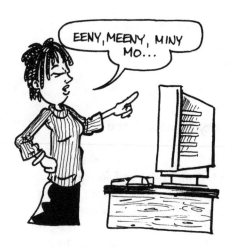

EENY, MEENY, MINY MO...

Chapter 5

Finding and Choosing Health Care

In This Chapter

➤ Using the Internet to help you choose or check on a doctor

➤ Learning about a particular hospital online

➤ Comparing health plans with online help

Managing your personal health care is a complicated challenge. Maybe you need to choose a new doctor because you moved, changed health plans, or need a particular specialty. Maybe you're curious about the credentials of your current doctor, or one who has been recommended to you. Maybe you need to locate a hospital that specializes in a certain surgery, or learn more about a medical test your doctor suggests. Or maybe you're trying to compare health plans. The Internet makes all of this possible—and faster and easier than you might expect. Web sites are springing up that let you investigate just about any health-care decision you need to make, and compare your options. This chapter shows you how to do it.

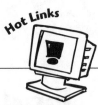

Your Guide to Choosing Quality Health Care

http://www.ahcpr.gov/consumer/qntool.htm

This exceptional guide from the Agency for Health Care Policy and Research (AHCPR) helps you figure out what's important to you, and then locate services that match your preferences. Choose either plain-text HTML or the nice-looking PDF format to read a comprehensive guide to making all those major health-care choices: health plan, doctor, treatments, hospital, long-term care, and health information on the Internet. AHCPR is the lead federal agency in charge of research on health-care quality, outcomes, cost, use, and access.

Doctor Checkup

Whether you're trying to learn about your current doctor or choosing a new one, the Internet is an amazing resource. Knowing that consumers want to take charge of their health care, many sites offering databases of physician information have popped up to make your research easy. You can find a gynecologist in a new city, learn if there have been any malpractice suits against your surgeon, or compare the qualifications of the pediatricians in your hometown.

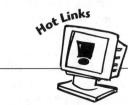

Choosing Quality Care

http://www.healthfinder.gov

Click **smart choices**, and then **choosing quality care** to see articles on how to choose a health plan, a primary-care professional, a hospital, a treatment, complementary therapy, long-term care, or choices for rural health selected by healthfinder.gov, a government gateway to reliable health information. Click **choosing primary care** for doctor-finders in many different specialties.

Good Doctor Checklist

The Agency for Health Care Policy and Research (AHCPR) offers the following "Quick Check for Quality" (http://www.ahcpr.gov/consumer/qntascii/qntdr.htm) for evaluating your doctor.

Look for a doctor who

➤ Is rated to give quality care.

➤ Has the training and background that meet your needs.

➤ Takes steps to prevent illness—for example, talks to you about quitting smoking.

➤ Has privileges at the hospital of your choice.

➤ Is part of your health plan, unless you can you afford to pay extra.

➤ Encourages you to ask questions.

➤ Listens to you.

➤ Explains things clearly.

➤ Treats you with respect.

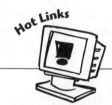

Hot Links

Give Your Doctor a Checkup

http://www.adventisthealthsocal.com/AHSC/MDs/1DocCheckup.html

This guide from Adventist Health/Southern California briefly explains the importance of a primary-care doctor and how to choose one.

Examining Your Doctor or Finding a New One

Your doctor knows everything about you, down to your athlete's foot, the findings of your last pelvic or prostate exam, and the mole on your left buttock. But what do you know about your doctor? Isn't it time to turn the tables? I'm not suggesting making your doctor put on one of those floppy examination wraps (although that *would* be interesting!), but wouldn't you like to know something more about his or her background?

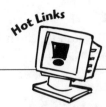

Hot Links

Finding Physician Credentials on the Internet

`http://www.healthcentral.com/news/column_schmalz.cfm?ID=16712`

Rochelle Perrine Schmalz, HealthCentral's medical librarian, covers in detail how and where to get background information on a physician by using online biographical directories; local and state medical societies and associations; hospital, health plan, and physician sites; and licensing and discipline resources. On the less-technical side, she tells you what you can learn from the certificates and diplomas on your doctor's office walls.

Even if you're perfectly happy with your doctor, you, like millions of Americans, might find yourself needing to choose a new physician because you move, change jobs, change health insurance, or need a specialist. How can you learn which doctors are available in the location or specialty you need, and can you learn enough to make an educated decision?

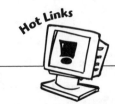

Hot Links

Doctors & Hospitals

`http://www.stayhealthy.com`

Under **Centers**, click **Doctors & Hospitals** for an array of links to sites that help you find a doctor, chiropractor, dentist, eye surgeon, dermatologist, or hospital.

You can learn a lot, and the following sites can help. Of course, finding a new doctor by reading a description online is a bit like reading personals ads—you can learn only so much, and you still need to meet to find out if you're *sympatico*. (But unlike most personals ads, at least you can count on the information you read as probably being the truth!) One caveat: Keeping a database of 600,000 licensed physicians up to date is close to impossible. Doctors move from one hospital or office affiliation to another. Don't let these sites be your only source of information. But they are wonderful places to start, and they might provide exactly the information you seek. The following sites provide tools for checking your doctor or finding a new one. All are free unless otherwise noted.

Health Pages

http://www.thehealthpages.com

"The Voice of the Health Care Consumer," Health Pages helps you find a physician, compare insurance plans, and explore health-care options (see Figure 5.1). This site has information on more than 500,000 physicians, 120,000 dentists, 300 managed care plans, Medicare plans, 6,000 hospitals, mammography clinics, fertility clinics, and maternity services. You can even rate your own doctor, dentist, or hospital by answering an 8-point survey, and your rating will be tabulated along with other patients' ratings and appear on the provider's page.

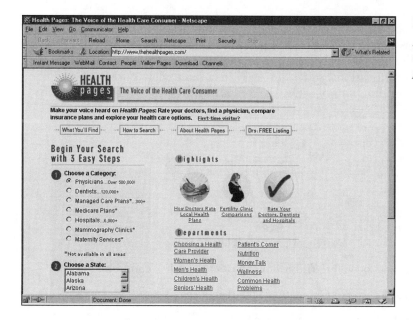

Figure 5.1

Health Pages helps you compare health-care providers.

AMA Physician Select

http://www.ama-assn.org/aps/amahg.htm

The American Medical Association's online "Physician Select" gives you access to the AMA's huge, comprehensive database of licensed physicians in the United States and its possessions, including more than 650,000 doctors of medicine (MD) and doctors of osteopathy or osteopathic medicine (DO). Search by location or specialty.

American Board of Medical Specialties (ABMS)

http://www.certifieddoctor.org

This service gives information about physicians who have been certified in one or more of the 24 specialties of the ABMS. Learn the doctor's board-certification status, location, contact information, hospital and health-plan affiliations, and links to physician and hospital Web pages.

AIM (Administrators in Medicine) DocFinder

`http://www.docboard.org/`

The Association of State Medical Board Executive Directors has links to state boards that license medical doctors, investigate complaints, and discipline those who violate the law. You need the correct spelling of the physician's first and last name or medical license number to locate information. Not every state is included here.

Medi-Net

`http://www.askmedi.com/`

"Medi-Net is a one-of-a-kind information delivery service that provides background information on every physician licensed to practice in the United States." A report on your physician, including medical school, residency training, American Board of Medical Specialties Certifications, states currently licensed in, licensure data, and records of sanctions or disciplinary actions taken against a physician's license, if any; it costs $14.75.

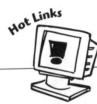

Hot Links

Medical Specialties

Looking for a particular specialty? The following doctor-finders can help:

➤ Chiropractor-Finder, `http://www.chiropractor-finder.com`

➤ Find a Dermatologist, `http://www.aad.org/findermi.html`

➤ LocateAnEyeDoc.Com, `http://patient.isrs.org/fndoctor/fndoctor.mv`

➤ Dental-Find, `http://www.dentalfind.com`

SearchPointe

`http://www.SearchPointe.com`

Search for a doctor (from a database of 650,000 physicians) or a chiropractor (see Figure 5.2). Information includes locations, credentials, disciplinary actions, professional background and credential verification. Some search services are free, such as a search for a physician in your area in the specialty you want. Other searches have a fee, such as $14 for a doctor's license and sanctions report.

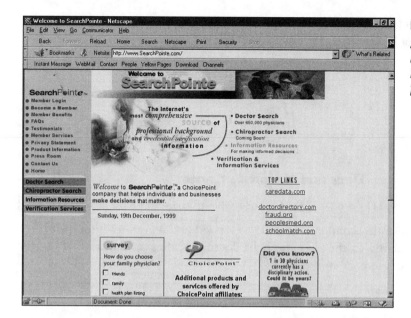

Figure 5.2
SearchPointe lets you find a doctor for free or do a background check for a fee.

HealthGrades.com

http://www.healthgrades.com

This site gives profiles on 600,000 physicians whose qualifications have been screened. It also rates 5,000 hospitals (by procedure or diagnosis) and 400 health plans, and has detailed guides on how to choose a hospital, physician, or health plan (click the topic of your choice under **Health Tools**).

Physician Search

http://www.bestdoctors.com/en/PhysicianSearch/index.asp

If you have a critical or complex medical situation, and finding the best doctor for the specialty you need is worth an investment, Best Doctors is a specialty-referral company that matches your case to the best doctors for $975. Best Doctors uses a database of only specialists who have been judged "best" by their peers. You can read a little about the service on the Web page, but you have to call to start the search. There's also a simple search function for getting the names of two physicians in the specialty and location you choose for $25.

Physician.com

http://www.physician.com

Under **For the Patient**, click **Doctor Find** to search by specialty and/or location, and obtain a doctor's name, address, licensure (with address of licensing board), medical school, and residencies. You can also look for a hospital or health insurance here. You can find a lot of information for free from this site.

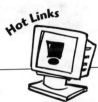

Docs and Hospitals Center

`http://www.stayhealthy.com/centers/docsandhospitals.cfm`

This site from Stayhealthy.com links to other reviewed and annotated sites for a variety of topics related to choosing the right doctor, locating a hospital, and obtaining valuable reference information.

Finding the Right Hospital

How do you know if a hospital you are considering is the best in your area for your needs? How do you know if it's worth traveling to a specialty hospital in another state for a particular procedure? The following sites not only rate hospitals, but also offer guides to making you an educated consumer. Check other categories in this chapter, because some of the sites that help you locate a doctor also compare hospitals.

HealthGrades.com

`http://www.healthgrades.com`

This site grades 5,000 hospitals (by procedure or diagnosis) and 400 health plans, and gives profiles on 600,000 physicians, 60,000 chiropractors, 300 fertility clinics, and 21,000 assisted-living residences. Be sure to read the guide on **How to Choose a Hospital** under the heading **Health Tools**.

All Hospitals Are Not Created Equal

`http://www.thehealthpages.com/articles/ar-hosps.html`

This article explains the different types of hospitals and the questions you should ask to choose a hospital where you will get the best treatment (see Figure 5.3). When you're done reading the article, enter your state and click **Review and Compare Hospitals** to see your options.

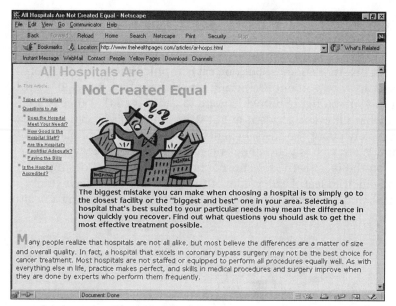

Figure 5.3

This Health Pages article explains how to evaluate a hospital.

Best Hospitals Finder

http://www.usnews.com/usnews/nycu/health/hosptl/tophosp.htm

The *U.S. News and World Report* ranks 6,299 hospitals by specialty to help you find the highest level of medical care. You can search for a hospital by region, or browse the top ranked hospitals.

HospitalDirectory.com

http://www.hospitaldirectory.com

Search by location and find out what hospitals are in that area. The only information given is address, phone number, and sometimes Web site.

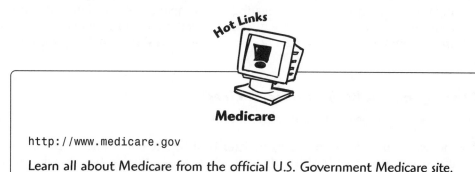

Hot Links

Medicare

http://www.medicare.gov

Learn all about Medicare from the official U.S. Government Medicare site.

71

Making Sense of Health Plans and Health Insurance

You hate to think about health insurance. But one catastrophic illness, accident, or extended hospital stay can wipe you out financially if you don't have the right health plan or insurance. How can you figure out which one to get? Given that there's no crystal ball to predict what illness or accident might strike, the best you can do is educate yourself extensively about the costs, benefits, and comparisons of plans available to you. The World Wide Web is your guide and partner. One of the ways the Internet can benefit you the most is the selection of helpful guides to choosing health care. There's so much to learn! The guides at the following sites teach you what you need to know, and some walk you through the process of choosing a health plan.

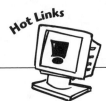

Assisted-Living Consumer Information and Resources

http://www.alfa.org/consumer.htm

This site from Assisted Living Federation of America presents a wealth of information about evaluating and choosing an assisted-living residence.

Choosing and Using a Health Plan

http://www.ahcpr.gov/consumer/hlthpln1.htm

The Agency for Health Care Policy and Research (AHCPR), a part of the U.S. Department of Health and Human Services, answers many of your questions about getting health-care insurance: investigating and comparing plans, getting the most from your plan, what to do if you're dissatisfied, getting a plan when you have pre-existing conditions, and choosing a doctor. This site gives solid advice, presented in a clear manner.

Checkup on Health Insurance Choices

http://www.ahcpr.gov/consumer/insuranc.htm

Another excellent guide from the Agency for Health Care Policy and Research, this site covers why you need health insurance, where to get it, what type is right for you, questions to ask, and a checklist for figuring out your best buy.

Health Insurance from Money.com

http://www.pathfinder.com/money/101/lessons/17/intro.html

"Even good coverage can have big loopholes." "The lowest premium isn't always the cheapest plan." These are two of the "top 10 things to know" from *Money* magazine's health-insurance lesson. Also learn the "basic flavors" of health insurance and the best strategies for saving money. Read the whole thing before buying health insurance.

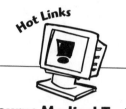

Hot Links

Laurus Medical Tests

http://www.laurushealth.com

Has your physician recommended a medical test that you don't fully understand? Click **Medical Tests** from the list on the left and learn about more than 200 common medical tests and procedures. Laurus gives plenty of information about each test, including why it is done, how it is done, how you prepare, even how it feels (with no sugar coating).

Your Complete Guide to Managed Care

http://www.thehealthpages.com/articles/ar-manag.html

"Everything you need to know about managed care, from the ABCs of HMOs to local plan comparisons." The Health Pages helps you choose the health-care coverage that suits you best. This site includes comprehensive "report cards" comparing the managed-care options available to you.

WellnessWeb Health Insurance Center

http://wellweb.com/INSURANCE/health_insurance_index.htm

Learn how to choose and use a health plan, including understanding your options, learning about benefits, comparing plans, evaluating quality, and getting the most from your plan.

Choosing a Health Plan

http://healthfinder.com/smartchoices/qualitycare/hcplans.htm

Healthfinder presents a long list of links to many reputable sites to learn about health insurance, managed care, Medicare, Medicaid, VA health care, and much more.

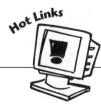

Surprise! Your Needs Aren't Covered

`http://onhealth.com/ch1/columnist/item,50809.asp`

Your employer switches insurance carriers, and suddenly one of your specialized medical needs is no longer covered. Health-care journalist Jan Greene tells you how to figure out what, if anything, you can do about it.

eHealthInsurance.com

`http://www.ehealthinsurance.com`

Shopping for health insurance? You can compare services and rates of different major medical insurance plans from a choice of leading companies, and then apply online (see Figure 5.4). Be sure to read FAQ to learn more about buying health insurance.

Figure 5.4

You can compare health insurance plans and apply online with eHealthInsurance.com.

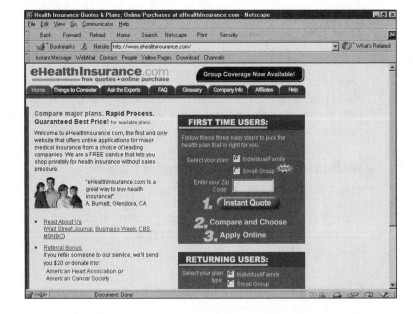

The Least You Need to Know

➤ You can check your doctor's credentials online or find a new doctor using location or specialty.

➤ You can find and compare hospitals at your location.

➤ Many helpful guides to choosing health insurance are available on the Web.

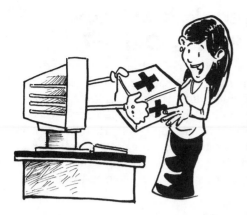

Chapter 6

Buying Medical Supplies Online

In This Chapter

➤ Protecting yourself when buying online

➤ Buying home health items online

➤ Finding disability devices online

➤ Purchasing vision care online

Of course you know that you can buy books, computers, and clothing online—but does it occur to you to buy your health-care and medical supplies by clicking your mouse? You can use the Internet to buy just about anything that doesn't have to be specially fitted or tested.

You need to comparison-shop to see if you actually find bargains online, but you certainly gain time and convenience. This chapter introduces you to some of the medical products you can buy online and where to shop. (If you're shopping for prescription drugs or herbs, please see Chapter 14, "Medications and Supplements.")

This chapter also gives you the scoop on how to cybershop safely, whatever you're buying.

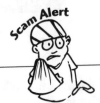

Overly Enthusiastic?

Don't buy on the recommendation of an enthusiastic user in a chat room or message board—unscrupulous companies sometimes plant messages that sound like the gushing of a satisfied user to draw buyers.

What Should You Know About Buying Online?

In many ways, buying medical supplies online follows the same rules, strategies, and cautions as buying anything else online. For a ton of information about buying online, read *The Complete Idiot's Guide to Online Shopping* by Preston Gralla. He tells you how to check out a site before buying, how to sniff out bargains, and how to find everything online: cars, clothes, computers, stocks, gifts, even apartments!

Safe Shopping

Whether you're buying a back support cushion, knee brace, nebulizer, or lift chair, follow these rules for safe buying:

➤ **Check out the company.** Ideally, you should be familiar with the company and its reputation. If that's not possible, make sure the company lists a real address and phone number.

➤ **Shop at secure sites.** A secure site encrypts confidential information. This means that it scrambles your personal information and credit card number before blasting it over cyberspace, so a hacker can't make any sense out of it. If the site you want to deal with is not secure, you might want to phone in your order instead.

➤ **Use a credit card.** As scary as it might be to give your credit card number to a stranger, this is safer than sending a check or cash—and no riskier than handing your credit card to a waiter. You can dispute a credit-card charge in case of a problem, such as the product not arriving. If you sent cash or check, the money's gone.

➤ **Figure total cost.** The advertised price of a product might be a bargain, but before you order, check out shipping charges, tax, and any other costs. You might not find this out until you fill your shopping cart and look at the total. (If you see a surprise that you don't like at that point, and you don't see a way to cancel the order, change all quantities to zero and update the order.)

➤ **Learn return policy.** Read the warranty and the company's policy for returning the item. Is there a time limit? Can you get your money back, or just exchange it?

Fraud Watch: Internet Tips

These tips from the National Fraud Information Center, a project of the National Consumers League (hotline: 1-800-876-7060), apply to all online shopping, not just medical products. Read more at http://www.fraud.org/internet/intset.htm.

Single Product Alert

Be wary of a site whose whole reason for being is to sell a single product. Check that this product is legitimate and your best choice before buying.

➤ **Do business with companies you know and trust.** Be sure you know who the company is and where it is physically located. Businesses operating in cyberspace might be in another part of the country or in another part of the world. Resolving problems with companies that are unfamiliar can be more complicated in long-distance or cross-border transactions.

➤ **Understand the offer.** Look carefully at the information about the products or services the company is offering, and ask for more information, if needed. A legitimate company will be glad to provide it; a fraudulent marketer won't. Be sure you know what is being sold, the total price, the delivery date, the return and cancellation policy, and the terms of any guaranty. The federal telephone and mail order rule, which also covers orders by computer, requires goods or services to be delivered by the promised time or, if none was stated, within 30 days. Print out the information so that you have documentation if you need it.

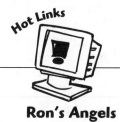

Ron's Angels

http://www.ronsangels.com/

When does a medical-sale site make the front page of *USA TODAY*? When models are selling their eggs. Starting bids are "$15,000 to $150,000 U.S. in $1,000.00 increments." This site wasn't chosen as a Hot Link because it's recommended—it's not. But a chapter on medical sales can't be complete without a glimpse into the *mondo bizarro* that answers the question, "How far will some people go?" By the way, this part didn't make the newspapers: Hunky guys are auctioning their sperm on the same site.

➤ **Check out the company's track record.** Ask your state or local consumer-protection agency if the company has to be licensed or registered, and with whom, and check to see if it is. You can also ask consumer agencies and the Better Business Bureau in your area about the company's complaint record. But keep in mind that fraudulent companies can appear and disappear quickly, especially in cyberspace, so lack of a complaint record is no guarantee that a company is legitimate.

➤ **Be careful to whom you give your financial or other personal information.** Don't provide your bank account numbers, credit card numbers, Social Security number, or other personal information unless you know the company is legitimate and the information is necessary for the transaction. Even with partial information, con artists can make unauthorized charges, deduct money from your account, and impersonate you to get credit in your name.

➤ **Take your time to decide.** Although there might be time limits for special offers, high-pressure sales tactics are often danger signs of fraud.

➤ **Be aware that there are differences between private sales and sales by a business.** All sorts of goods and services are sold or traded by individuals through unsolicited emails, newsgroups postings, chat room discussions, Web auctions, and online classified advertisements. While most people are honest, your legal rights against the seller may not be the same as with a business, and you could have difficulty pursuing your complaint if the merchandise is misrepresented, defective, or never delivered.

➤ **You may be better off paying by credit card than with a check, cash, or money order, as long as you know with whom you're doing business.** When you use your credit card for a purchase and there is a problem, you have the right to notify your card issuer that you are disputing the charge, and you don't have to pay it while your dispute is being investigated. It's easier to resolve a problem if you haven't already paid. Also, unless you are purchasing through a secured site (preferably one that's using the new Secured Encryption Technology), it might be safer to provide your payment information by phone or mail rather than online.

➤ **Don't judge reliability by how nice or flashy a Web site might seem.** Anyone can create, register, and promote a Web site; it's relatively easy and inexpensive. And just like any other forms of advertising, you can't assume that someone has screened and approved it.

➤ **Know that people in cyberspace may not always be what they seem.** Someone who is sharing a "friendly" tip about a money-making scheme or great bargain in a chat room or on a bulletin board might have an ulterior motive: to make money. And sometimes those friendly people turn out to be crooks!

➤ **Know that unsolicited email violates computer etiquette and is often used by con artists.** It also violates most agreements for Internet service. Report *spamming*, as unsolicited email is called, to your online or Internet service provider.

➤ **Don't download programs to see pictures, hear music, or get other features from Web sites you're not familiar with.** You could unwittingly download a virus that wipes out your computer files or even hijacks your Internet service, reconnecting you to the Net through an international phone number, resulting in enormous phone charges.

Medical Supply Megasites

Before you go in search of a site that specializes in the category you want to buy, take a look at the following megasites. They offer an enormous cross-section of health and medical supplies. Maybe you can find everything you want in one place!

MedQue.com

`http://www.medque.com`

Doorknob turners, zipper pulls, raised toilet seats, breast pumps, back supports, cervical collars, ostomy pouches, nebulizers, wheelchair ramps—these are just a few of the products you'll find for sale at this megastore. "The largest online medical supply store" sells thousands of products (see Figure 6.1). MedQue.com also has links to related medical content sites.

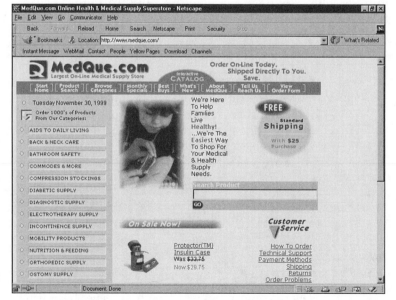

Figure 6.1

MedQue.com sells all categories of medical supplies.

Rx.com

http://www.Rx.com/

Click **Nonprescription Products**. Under **Healthcare Supplies**, choose from braces, wraps, and supports; diabetes management; first aid; home health care (including backrests, bath seats, canes, crutches, nebulizers, and home test kits); incontinence; patient aids; smoking cessation; and sports medicine.

PlanetRx

http://www.planetrx.com/

Click **Medical Supplies** in the area marked **The Store**, and then the product category you want: appliances, bandages and splints, diabetic care, first aid, home assistance (including canes and bathroom safety), home test kits (including HIV, blood pressure, lung function, and pregnancy tests), or incontinence.

SelfCare

http://www.selfcare.com/

This site includes five stores where you can buy nonprescription remedies, medicinal supplies, alternative-therapy devices (such as light therapy and acupressure tools), orthopedic support (for neck, spine, and legs), and items for a healthy home (analyzers, monitors, bedding systems, mobility aids, massage, whirlpools, and purification appliances).

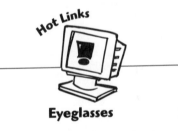

Hot Links

Eyeglasses

http://ophthalmology.about.com/health/ophthalmology/msubeyeglass.htm

Night driving, eyeglass anatomy, sunglass smarts—before you buy your next pair, learn all about eyeglasses in this array of interesting articles assembled by About.com.

Vision Care

You've been eating your carrots, but your vision still hasn't improved. Never mind, eyeglasses are not only functional, they're in style. And if you don't want an object propped on your nose, contact lenses are a super solution.

As long as you have a current prescription, you can buy eyeglasses and contact lenses online; and you can learn plenty about vision, eye care, and eyewear on the Web.

Contacts

New to contact lenses? If you have never been fitted for lenses, you can't just order them. Contacts not only have to have the correct vision prescription, they also must fit your eyes correctly and comfortably. A "live" eye-care professional has to examine your eyes, fit you for lenses, and train you how to insert and remove them.

If you already wear contact lenses, however, and your prescription is up to date, you can order lenses online. The following are some of the sites that offer this service.

CLE Contact Lenses

`http://contactlensexpress.com/`

This site sells all types of contact lenses (sealed from the manufacturer) and also provides information about contacts and links to medical sites. "Our team of eye care professionals are anxious to answer any questions you may have concerning eye health, diseases, surgery, exercises, low vision, contact lenses, eye glasses, and more."

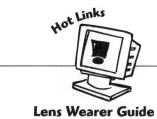

Lens Wearer Guide

`http://0clecontactlenses.com/guide.html`

This superb guide from CLE Contact Lenses explains everything you need to know about how to clean, wear, insert, remove, and care for your contact lenses, including photographs.

Lens4Me

`http://www.lens4me.com/`

This Internet contact-lens source sells contacts and sunglasses, and offers plenty of free information. Click **Eye Advice** to read helpful tips for a variety of common eye problems with contact lenses, written in a peppy, friendly style.

Glasses

Buying eyeglasses online gives you plentiful frame and tint options and saves you time. But realize that even if your prescription is correct, your glasses might not fit your face properly, and no one will adjust them for you. (Don't expect your local optical retailer to adjust online-purchased glasses!) It's your call!

Focusers

`www.focusers.com/`

From this site you can buy prescription eyeglasses, reading glasses, and sunglasses after viewing photos of traditional and trendy frames. You'll enjoy their entertainingly overwritten descriptions, such as "suitable only for women who have cultivated an exquisite cachet...despite their brilliance in color, they carry with them the muted mystique of a femme fatale in a black-and-white Fellini film."

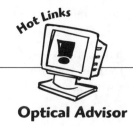

Hot Links

Optical Advisor

http://www.opticaladvisor.com/

"Optical Advisor helps you look your best, see your best, and get the best value when purchasing eyewear." Learn about eyeglasses, contact lenses, optical surgery, and more from this informative site. Be sure to click the unbiased **Pros and Cons of Purchasing Eyewear Online**.

Disability Devices

Here's where the World Wide Web really shines. If you or a loved one has a disability that restricts mobility or vision, particularly, you can shop online for just about everything you need.

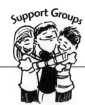

Support Groups

Web Corners

http://pages.prodigy.net/disabilitymall/wcpps.htm

This support jump site from the Disability and Medical Resource Mall offers links to pen pals, forums, bulletin boards, chat rooms, and other support resources for people with disabilities.

Majors Medical Supply

http://www.majorsmedical.com/

This site sells wheelchairs, scooters, home care items, lift chairs/recliners, and products for pediatrics, respiratory disease, diabetes, and colostomy. A unique service is customizing rehab wheelchairs for people from 18 pounds to 800 pounds.

Disability & Medical Resource Mall

http://www.disabilitystore.com

This directory features "disability and medical products, resources, and services with over 2,500 links including over 400 companies." Founded and developed by the disabled, this site provides information on products and resources available to the disabled, handicapped, physically challenged, elderly, caregivers, and health-care professionals and providers (see Figure 6.2).

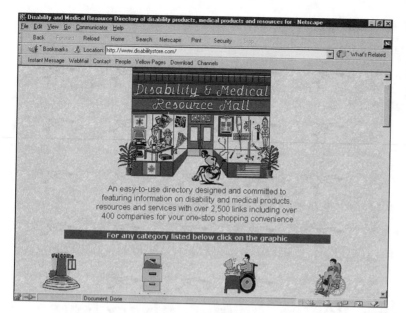

Figure 6.2

The Disability & Medical Resource Mall links to thousands of resources for persons with disabilities.

The Boulevard

http://www.blvd.com/

This is a jump site for people with disabilities and health-care professionals to learn about an amazing variety of products and services, including wheelchair-accessible vacations, van conversions, adaptive clothing, home management, and adaptive computer equipment. If you need it, this site lists companies that have it.

Adaptive Computer Products

http://www.eskimo.com/~jlubin/disabled/computers.htm

Computer hardware and software have been adapted so that a person with any disability can use them easily and productively. This helpful site offers links to not only adaptive computer products, programs, and services, but also to articles explaining the different technologies.

Independent Living Aids

http://www.independentliving.com/

"CAN-DO products—to make everyday living easier!" This site offers a variety of aids for the visually handicapped: watches, calculators, telephones, cooking tools, magnifiers, reading machines, sound amplifiers, personal care products, and more.

Independent Living Products

http://www.ilp-online.com/

"Turn Can't Into Can!" This catalog of assistive devices helps people with physical limitations maintain their independence. These products help people bathe, dress, eat, use the toilet, walk, get in and out of a bed or chair, and enjoy hobbies and recreation.

Med-Sell

http://www.medsell.com/

"Your resource guide for new and previously owned medical equipment, assistive devices and services." Med-Sell helps you buy and sell used medical equipment: wheelchair-equipped vans, scooters, hospital beds, sleep-apnea machines, TENS units, ramps, and much more. This site also features articles and links to other disability-related sites.

Who Knows What You're Buying? Privacy Issues

If you want privacy, you'd better tuck your hair under a cap, attach a fake moustache, shop at the mall, and pay cash. Shopping online is like going on a buying spree accompanied by a caravan of reporters. Everywhere you go and everything you buy can be tracked.

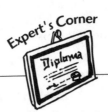

You're Not Alone

"On the Internet, you're never really alone. And nothing you do online is private. Everything that you do when you visit a site can be tracked—not just what you buy, but what products you look at, how long you spend on the site, what you read on the site, what site you visited before visiting the shopping site, and where you went next."

—Preston Gralla, author of *The Complete Idiot's Guide to Online Shopping* (Macmillan, 1999).

Online merchants like to learn what you look at and what you buy so that they can better serve you—and themselves, of course. Reputable sites keep this information to themselves, or at least give you the chance to say you don't want your information passed along. But realize that a site can make a pretty penny by selling that information to direct marketers. To minimize the chance of that happening to you, ask these questions before you buy:

➤ **What is the privacy policy?** How will this site use the information it collects about you? A reputable site will state its privacy policy clearly (and post it where you can find it). If you don't see it, ask for it. If you don't get an answer—or don't like the answer you get—shop somewhere else.

➤ **Does this site adhere to rules from a privacy watchdog?** Certain privacy watchdogs issue seals to sites that honor their policies. For example, sites that display the TRUSTe seal agree to adhere to TRUSTe's privacy principles and allow to an "oversight" process. Read about how this benefits you at http://www.truste.org/users/.

➤ **Can you just say no?** If the site does "share" or "make available to select vendors" (that means "sell") its information, does it have an "opt-out" policy? This means that you can say you don't want your information sold, and they agree not to do it.

➤ **What does that small print say?** Read every word of the order form and order information. If the site asks if you want to be informed about special offers or information, say no or uncheck the box. Look for every opportunity to let them know that you don't want this order to be the beginning of a one-sided pen-pal experience.

➤ **Why do I have to tell you this?** If the order form asks questions that have nothing to do with your order, like your age or income, don't answer. Some sites have an asterisk (*) indicating the questions that absolutely have to be answered. Ignore the others.

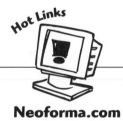

Neoforma.com

http://www.neoforma.com/home/

In the market for your own MRI machine? How about a colonoscope? Or maybe a used plastic surgery table? This site is a "global health-care marketplace" that sells and auctions new and used medical equipment. Okay, it's aimed at hospitals, not home consumers like you, but in case you might be interested in setting up your own E.R....

The Least You Need to Know

➤ You can buy just about any type of health-care or medical supply online.

➤ Follow your head (rather than your hunger for a bargain) when evaluating whether to buy from a particular site.

➤ The World Wide Web is a superb source of disability devices of all types.

➤ Check a site's privacy policy before disclosing personal information.

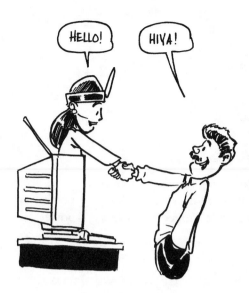

HELLO!

HIYA!

Chapter 7

You and Your Doc: A Partnership

In This Chapter

➤ Creating a partnership between you and your doctor

➤ Conferring with your doctor about what you're learning online

➤ The future of medicine and the Internet

➤ Making use of the Internet to enhance your interactions with your physician

➤ Keeping your medical history online

The computer has transformed just about every aspect of how medical professionals do their jobs. A whole new world is opening—a world of information and communication—and you're the beneficiary.

Although patients used to have to be, well, *patient* waiting for their physicians to feed them morsels of knowledge, now patients are educating themselves with mouse clicks and modems. There are ways to use your Internet research that enhance your relationship with your doctor and speed your treatment, and other ways that interfere with both. This chapter helps you accomplish the former!

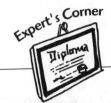

Fact Versus Wisdom

"Don't believe everything you read on the Internet. There is a difference between information and knowledge, between facts and wisdom. Ask your doctor to help you sort through what you find on the Web. Indeed, knowledge is power, but the challenge is using it wisely!"

—Holly Atkinson, M.D., Editor, *HealthNews*

Ask Your M.D. First

The Internet has opened possibilities that neither patients nor doctors could have imagined just a couple of decades ago. You can read consumer medical sites (see the recommended "Medical Super Sites" in this book), or you can even go to the source and read the medical journals and professional sites where doctors get their own information.

You might even get so light-headed over this cornucopia of information that you wonder if you can bypass the doctor's appointment. Who needs Dr. Doc when the Internet tells you what's wrong with you and what to do about it?

Stop!

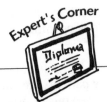

Mouse Checkup No Substitute

"Is the annual checkup a thing of the past? Not likely. Proper diagnosis and treatment can't happen with the click of the mouse. It's a newer, faster way to learn about pre-existing conditions, but it's not a substitute for a trip to the doctor's office. And be wary—you can't believe everything you read."

—Robert Min, M.D., Clinical Director of The Vein Treatment Center, New York City (www.veintreatmentcenter.com)

There are a billion reasons why you shouldn't take any advice or try any treatment from the Internet without consulting with your physician about it first. Try the following reasons on for size:

➤ Your physician knows the intimate details of your condition and how you have responded to other treatments.

➤ Your physician knows your medical history.

➤ Just because you have a particular condition doesn't mean a particular therapy is right for you—there are many more variables than just the name of the condition.

➤ Your physician knows what other conditions you have, what other medications you are taking, and what therapeutic interactions you might expect from combining these with a new treatment.

➤ Much of what you read on the Internet is hogwash.

➤ Your medical degree is sadly lacking.

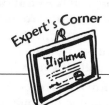

Dialog with Your Doc

"The Internet has done wonders for the medical community, creating a new way for doctors and patients to communicate with each other. Before you use medical information found online to treat or diagnose an illness, discuss online findings with your family physician. And don't be afraid to tell him or her that you located the information online. Physicians welcome educated patients, especially when they use the information they find online to open up a dialogue with the physician. Use information found on the Internet as a supplement to advice and treatment provided by a medical professional."

—Raj Lakhanpal, M.D., founder and president of HealthAtoZ.com (www.healthAtoZ.com)

How to Talk to Your Doctor About What You're Learning

You're learning some great information about your condition and treatments options. You can't wait to tell your doctor what you've found! Slow down—educated patients might be new to your doctor, and you need to approach your physician with soft shoes rather than combat boots.

Be careful not to appear as if you're playing doctor yourself. If you run into your doctor's office and announce, "Hey, Doc, I've found the cure for my cancer right here at www.scamcancerscamcurescam.com!" your doctor will suspect that you shouldn't be making any of your own decisions (and dread your next visit). Ditto if you insist on any particular treatment or surgery based on what you read on a Web site.

For a more effective approach that will please rather than pester your physician, use the following guidelines:

➤ **Acknowledge that your doctor contributes to your knowledge and is your guide in your search for information.** For example, start by saying, "When you gave me two treatment options, I decided to learn more about each one of them" or "Your explanation of how my disease is progressing made me want to explore some patient guides from reputable medical sites."

➤ **Show that you know how to find credible sites.** Explain your use of the PILOT method. (No, the doctor won't recognize the *name* unless he or she has read either this book or *The Complete Idiot's Guide to Online Health and Fitness*, because Shannon Entin and I invented it. You'll have to explain the steps.) Your doctor sees so many patients who fall for quack sites that he or she will be impressed that you know how to evaluate a site for credibility.

➤ **Let your doctor personalize and enhance the research you've done.** Ask questions like, "Now that I've got more background, I have some more questions for you" and "Is this a treatment you would recommend, given my particular medical history and condition?"

➤ **Ask for recommended sites.** Ask your doctor which sites have the best patient information to help you understand your condition or treatment. (This is also a subtle way to find out if your doctor knows much about the Internet. If not, this book would be a great gift!)

➤ **Ask for homework.** Ask, "What would you suggest that I learn about before my next visit?"

Occasionally you'll find doctors who don't like patients doing their own research on the Web. They might feel threatened because they, personally, don't use online resources, and they don't plan to get up to speed anytime soon. Others enjoy the role of Dr. God and would rather have you ask questions than find the answers yourself. If your doctor resembles either of these descriptions, it might be time to question whether you want to stick with this doctor.

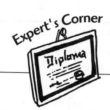

Some Docs Don't

"Some doctors don't appreciate any meaningful involvement of patients in their own care and view patients that do their own research as troublesome. Perhaps they feel threatened that the patient doesn't simply accept their word without questioning. If that's the case with your doctor, you've got to ask yourself whether you're seeing the right one."

—Timothy B. McCall, M.D., internist and author of *Examining Your Doctor: A Patient's Guide To Avoiding Harmful Medical Care* (Citadel Press, 1995)

Your Physician and Your Printout

Don't just tell your doctor, "I read it on the Internet." Bring hard copies of the information you want to discuss with your doctor. Be sure to identify each printout with the URL and the name of the site. Make copies that you can leave with your physician *if* he or she requests them to look up the sites later.

Be realistic about the amount of information you expect to cover. Your physician doesn't have the time (or inclination!) to swim through an ocean of printouts. You might separate your printouts into a very small "ask doc about this" pile and a larger "background" pile in case you need to refer back to something else you learned.

Organize everything carefully. Bring a short, carefully prepared list of questions for your physician and a notebook or clipboard for recording the answers.

Do not antagonize your doctor by wheeling in a wagon-full of printouts and offering to leave them with your doctor overnight!

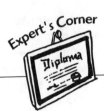

Sales Pitch Alert

"There is a lot of good medical information available on the Internet, but realize that some online medical 'information' is really disguised marketing of products that at best may not work, but may even be harmful. Most doctors cannot keep up with all these products, and may not be able to either defend or give good reasons to reject them. So be wary if the information is accompanied by a sales pitch."

—Larry Kassman, M.D., F.A.C.E.P.

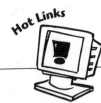

Medical Dictionaries

If your physician or the Web site you're reading uses medical terminology that you don't understand, look up that word in an online medical dictionary. Familiarize yourself with both of the following, and use the one that helps you most:

➤ `http://www.medicinenet.com` Click **dictionary** at the top. It's easy to find the word you want because it's in an alphabetical list—you don't have to be able to spell it yourself.

➤ `http://www.intelihealth.com` Scroll down the right side until you get to **Health Resources**. Click **Merriam Webster Medical Dictionary** for 40,000 medical words and definitions. You have to spell the word correctly.

The best-case scenario is this: Your doctor is thrilled by your Web exploration, praises you for making his or her work that much easier, says "Wow" and takes some notes while reading your pet printout, and nods approvingly at your conclusions.

But please be prepared to learn that your conclusions were wrong. The amazing cure you thought you found might be a sham, or an experimental therapy not proven safe or effective. The convincing article that got you excited about an herbal product might be advertising in disguise and unsubstantiated by any evidence. The therapy you read about on several reputable sites might be wrong for you personally, because of another condition or medication that you're taking.

Let your physician guide you to information that is more appropriate. Use his or her suggestions to make you a smarter surfer!

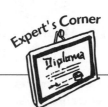

Expert's Corner

Doctors Use the Internet

"Physicians are increasingly using the World Wide Web to find medical information—and the quality of that information is getting better all the time. Email, telemedicine, sharing medical records, electronic prescribing, and other technologies made possible by the Internet will increasingly change the way medicine is practiced."

—Timothy B. McCall, M.D., internist and author of *Examining Your Doctor: A Patient's Guide To Avoiding Harmful Medical Care* (Citadel Press, 1995)

The Physician, the Patient, and the Internet

In a few years, most physicians and patients probably will be interacting via the Internet much more than they are now. The following possibilities—rare today—will be commonplace in the near future:

➤ If you have an ongoing illness and you want to ask your doctor a routine question or report on reactions to a treatment, you'll be able to communicate via email and maybe skip an office visit.

➤ Physicians will post articles on their Web sites. Their sites will include links to reputable medical sites for additional information.

➤ Your medical record will be computerized and accessible by all your health professionals (even if they're at different locations).

➤ Your doctor will teleconference with specialists in other countries.

➤ Your doctors will email you information about your diagnosis and/or medical condition, and will send you specific Web sites with information about your condition.

Some doctors are ahead of the pack and are already doing some of these activities. You can expect many more to join them soon. (You can also expect some to resist—doctors don't like change any more than the rest of us.)

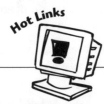

New Technologies in Medicine and Medical Journals

http://www.bmj.com/content/vol319/issue7220/

The prestigious *British Medical Journal* devotes a whole issue (November 13, 1999) to the theme of how new technologies will affect medicine. Read an array of articles on hospitals of the future, new technologies, and informatics. It's all online here, and you can choose to read abridged text or full text.

Email and Your M.D.

Forty percent of patients in a University of Michigan study (http://www.med.umich.edu/choices/intel.html) regularly use email, but only 14 percent of them have used it to communicate with their doctors. Seventy percent of patients surveyed—including those who don't use email yet—said that they would like to have email communication with their health-care provider. Eighty-three percent of the patients' physicians considered email a good way to answer patients' non-urgent medical questions, but only 27 percent currently use email to communicate with patients. Can you see the direction we're heading?

Are you lucky enough to have a physician who communicates with you by email? If not, bring up the subject at your next visit. Ask your physician, "Do you use email? How do you feel about using it to communicate with patients?"

Use the following guidelines for emailing your physician to help you use the system most effectively, protect your privacy, and avoid annoying or frustrating your doctor. And if your physician does not offer email access, you might have the edge in convincing him or her if you suggest that you'll follow these guidelines.

➤ Never use email for urgent messages. Call 911 if it's an emergency, or call your doctor if you have urgent needs.

➤ Ask your physician what response time to expect. If the normal response time has elapsed for an email you've sent, follow up by phone.

➤ Ask your physician who else reads his or her email, such as a nurse or office assistant. Does someone else read or process email after hours or during vacations?

➤ Ask what information your physician would like you to include in all emails, such as a patient ID number or date of birth. Avoid sending Social Security numbers via email.

➤ Use email for things like renewing prescriptions, checking on appointment times, or following up after a visit. Discuss other uses with your physician.

➤ Do not use email for topics that should be discussed face-to-face, such as a complicated set of symptoms.

➤ Do not use email to communicate about sensitive topics, such as HIV status.

➤ Treat any email you send as if it were an addition to your medical record—it will probably end up there.

(Many thanks to the American Medical Informatics Association at www.amia.org for assisting in compiling these guidelines.)

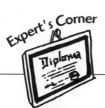

Doctor/Patient Email

"Email has the potential to improve both the quality and efficiency of health-care delivery. I think more and more patients and physicians will begin taking advantage of the ease and convenience of email as we begin this next century."

—Steven J. Katz, M.D., M.P.H., Associate Professor in the Departments of Medicine and Health Management and Policy at the University of Michigan

Web Info from Your M.D.

Your physician or his or her hospital or clinic might already have a Web site with patient information posted. Ask your doctor for the URL, and explore the Web site. Is it basically a promotional site, designed to bring in patients? Or does it provide a service for current patients by offering information and direction? Provide feedback to your doctor about how it could be more useful to you and other patients.

If your physician is not personally involved in a Web site, he or she should still be able to point you to the best ones where you can get good information on your condition. If this isn't already available, suggest that a patient handout with the best sites listed and annotated would be a tremendous benefit. It would also save the physician time by not having to repeat the same information to everyone who asks.

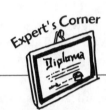

Information Prescriptions

"What patients and families want most is information from their own physician, whether that is by talking with them, handouts, or the Internet. What physicians must do is to write 'information prescriptions' for their patients and families that come from authoritative health information sources on the Internet. This will make for a more knowledgeable and hopefully healthier patient and family."

—Donna D'Alessandro, M.D., Assistant Professor of Pediatrics, Children's Hospital of Iowa, http://www.generalpediatrics.com, http://www.vh.org, and http://www.vnh.org

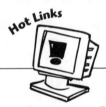

Patient Resource Center

http://www2.ahima.org/consumer/index.html

What's in your health record? Who owns it? Can you get access to it? What steps can you take to ensure confidentiality? This practical guide from the American Health Information Management Association answers these questions and more. Click **Patient Health Record Forms** to download forms you can fill out to keep your own health record.

Your Medical History Online

How many times have you dug through notes and old calendars to figure out when you had your last Pap smear or annual exam? Did you feel like a fool when your doctor asked when your hot flashes started? Are the results of your cholesterol test meaningless because you don't remember what they were the last time? Do you hate having to remember all your medications every time you have an office visit?

Wouldn't it be nice to have your whole medical history (and that of your spouse and kids) online? Hospitals and medical offices are gearing up to accomplish that, and several Web sites are offering it to you now. Enter your information once, and it's there. Forever.

No more giving the same information over and over again because the health professional can't find it in the thick folder of papers recording every office visit, prescription, and phone call in dozens of different handwritings. No problem if you switch doctors or move to a different city.

There is, however, a problem: privacy. If you're storing your information on a Web site, you want easy access to it. But the easier it is for you to access, the easier it is for other people to access, too. There's the rub.

And suppose your medical history is on your HMO's, doctor's, or hospital's computer. How many people have access to it, and for what reason, and how many hoops do they have to jump through to get at your records? What safeguards are in place?

This is a giant issue. The Department of Health and Human Services (HHS) has proposed a rule for "Standards for Privacy of Individually Identifiable Health Information" to protect the privacy of your personal health information stored in a computer or transmitted electronically (see `http://www.jhita.org/medical.htm`). Other rules, laws, and standards will race to keep up with the technological possibilities. Until that gets ironed out, be very careful about who gets your confidential information.

The following Web sites offer you the opportunity to store your personal medical record online and take pains to protect your privacy. Read their posted privacy policies first.

MyHealthRecord

`http://my.webmd.com/my_health_record`

WebMDHealth lets you store your medical information online, then print it out to carry to your next doctor's appointment (see Figure 7.1). Keep track of illnesses, allergies, medications, reactions, symptoms, and physicians.

Figure 7.1

MyHealthRecord from WebMD is your online vault for personal and family medical information.

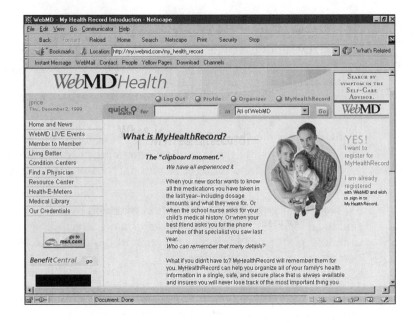

PersonalMD.com

http://www.PersonalMD.com/

Click **Medical Records**. You can include records of visits to the doctor or hospital, lab results, X-ray reports, EKGs, medications, allergies, childhood illnesses and shots, "and any information that can help your physician give you the best treatment possible."

HealthAtoZ E-Mate

http://www.healthatoz.com/

Click **HealthAtoZ E-Mate** to enter or view health and immunization records, your doctor's phone number, directions to your local hospital, your medications, refills, and supplements, and to schedule email reminders of upcoming health events.

iVillage allHealth.com

http://www.allhealth.com/

Click **Confidential Medical Records** to register for **My Health Records**, where you can store your medical information and history, including prescriptions, allergies, emergency contacts, tests, surgeries, and more.

The Least You Need to Know

➤ You can be an active partner in your health care by discussing your online discoveries with your doctor.

➤ In the near future, doctors and patients will commonly use the Internet to exchange and store information.

➤ Storing your personal medical information online is handy, but be careful about how your privacy is protected.

Part 3
Staying Well

If you're feeling well, the chapters in Part 3 will help you stay that way. And if you need some medical information that doesn't warrant a trip to the doctor, these chapters provide it for you. (Of course, if you really should see a doctor but are trying to find an answer in this book instead, expect a wagging finger, print style!)

Special chapters in Part 3 focus on the special health concerns of women, men, and children to help you find the kind of information that will keep you and your loved ones healthy. A distinctive chapter on sexuality shows you how to find sexual information that helps you enhance and protect your health and wellness without getting hijacked by sleazy sites.

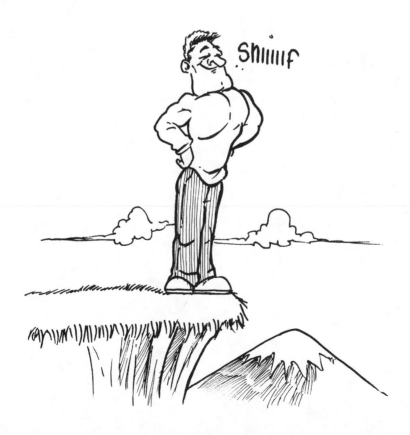

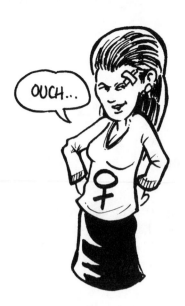

OUCH...

Women's Health

Women account for 52 percent of the United States population, yet they make 75 percent of the health care decisions and spend 65 percent of health care dollars—about $500 billion a year. One in three women use the Internet to get medical information, compared to one in four men. So you can see why health Web sites (and their advertisers) are eager to attract women.

The result is a profusion of women's health information blooming on just about every health and medical site, including our Medical Super Sites. Most have women's health centers, and all have information about specific conditions of concern to women.

You could, however, get lost taking the myriad paths offered you, so this chapter shows you the best highways and byways to women's health information. (If you're looking for a particular topic and don't find it in this chapter, check out the women's issues in Chapter 10, "Sexuality;" Chapter 12, "Getting Unhooked: Fighting Addictions;" Chapter 20, "Cancer;" Chapter 23, "Heart Disease;" and Chapter 25, "Osteoporosis.")

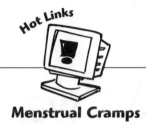

Menstrual Cramps

`http://bodymatters.com/bodymatters/cramps.html`

Fifty percent of women suffer from menstrual cramps (the medical term is dysmenorrhea), and half of these have cramps so severe that they have to take time off from work or school. This article from Body Matters, sponsored by Tampax, discusses what it feels like, what you can do about it, and other conditions that might be causing or worsening your cramps.

Starting Here: General Women's Health Sites

Superb sites abound with every women's health topic you can imagine. Get a general overview of women's health, or look up particular conditions at the following exceptional sites.

Content Sites

Content sites offer information written either specifically for the site or in association with another resource. The following are some favorite content sites for women's health.

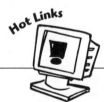

The Museum of Menstruation and Women's Health

`http://www.mum.org`

You've got to see this one! The Museum of Menstruation and Women's Health is a lively virtual museum tracking the history of tampons, menstrual cups, douches, washable pads, and sponges. View the first Kotex ad from 1921. Read about the "Lister's Towel" pad from the 1890s that never caught on. View the 1928 *Vanity Fair* ad for the "Sanitary Step-In"—underpants with a rubber crotch.

National Women's Health Information Center

`http://www.4woman.gov/`

This exceptional site from the Department of Health and Human Services' Office on Women's Health offers an array of Federal and other women's health information resources. You can search by health topic for remarkably clear and well-written information, or read almost 200 FAQs on various diseases, injuries, conditions, and other topics.

Women's Health Center

`http://www.wellweb.com/women/women.htm`

Wellness Web's Women's Health Center is warm, inviting, and educational (see Figure 8.1). Its articles cover screening tests, diseases, pregnancy, and more.

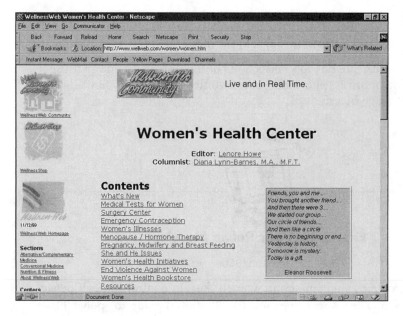

Figure 8.1

The Women's Health Center from Wellness Web offers information with a community atmosphere.

HealthAtoZ.com

`http://www.healthatoz.com`

HealthAtoZ.com has several "wellness centers" of special interest to women: Expectant Moms, Happy Parenting, and Women's Health. Read peppy articles about all issues related to women's health, including "Choosing Your Gynecologist" and "Staying Healthy in a Man's World."

iVillage Women's Health

`http://www.allhealth.com/womens/`

This women's health center from allHealth, the health site from iVillage ("the women's network") has articles, expert Q&As, news stories, message boards, chats, and special events for women. The site has a feeling of community.

Women's Health Interactive

`http://www.womens-health.com/`

This site offers interactive learning centers about a variety of women's health issues, such as gynecological concerns, headaches, depression, menopause, and natural health. Under each category you find a variety of topics, each of which presents a wealth of information after you click the components.

Her Health

`http://www.thriveonline.com/health/herhealth/index.html`

ThriveOnline's Her Health site has special sections on menopause, endometriosis, incontinence, and osteoporosis, plus many other women's medical topics, advice from experts, and message boards.

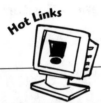

Hot Links

Exercising Your Pelvic Muscles

`http://www.niddk.nih.gov/health/urolog/uibcw/exerc/exerc.htm`

Bladder control problems are common in women. Regain control through pelvic muscle exercises, also called Kegel exercises. This illustrated guide to "pelvic fitness in minutes a day" from the National Kidney and Urologic Diseases Information Clearinghouse shows you exactly what to do.

Jump Sites

"Jump sites" don't have their own content; they provide links to other sites. The best ones offer reviewed links, which means they screen these links for credibility.

Society for Women's Health Research

`http://www.womens-health.org/factsheet.html`

This site from the Society for Women's Health Research is an excellent resource for links to reputable medical organizations that offer content information about women's health topics, from battering to osteoporosis. You also get interesting statistics and other facts.

Women's Health

`http://www.nytimes.com/specials/women/whome/resources.html`

The New York Times On the Web line offers an annotated guide to more than 100 reputable Web sites on women's health—a terrific resource. Links are categorized by General Health, Aging, AIDS, and specific conditions and diseases.

Women's Health Center

`http://www.stayhealthy.com/centers/women.cfm`

This superb women's health center from Stayhealthy.com connects you to a variety of reviewed, rated, and annotated links. Categories include endometriosis, hysterectomy, infertility, menopause, menstruation, pelvic inflammatory disease, pregnancy, reproductive health, and much more (see Figure 8.2).

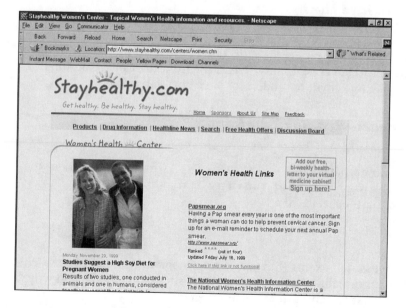

Figure 8.2

Stayhealthy.com's Women's Health Center has links to many women's wellness topics.

Screening Tests

Although none of us likes to imagine getting a disease like cancer, many types are curable or manageable if caught early. Regular screening tests while you're healthy can be essential tools for survival, and the World Wide Web teaches you all about them.

Pap Smears

What an ugly name for such a beneficial and simple procedure! This test detects precancerous changes in cells in the cervix. Cervical cancer usually develops slowly, so if abnormalities are detected early, they can be treated before they develop into cancer.

The College of American Pathologists recommends that every woman who is 18 or older or who is sexually active have an annual Pap smear, including women who are past menopause. Learn more about this screening test from the following sites.

Pap Smears

http://www.wellweb.com/women/papsmear.htm

What is a Pap smear, why should you get one, and what should you expect? This Wellness Web site presents 10 questions and answers about Pap smears, courtesy of the National Cancer Institute.

Annual Pap Smears Save Lives

http://www.papsmear.org/

"Scheduling and having a Pap smear every year is one of the most important things a woman can do to help prevent cervical cancer." This site from the College of American Pathologists lets you schedule email reminders for your next Pap smear.

Abnormal Pap Smears—Reading Your Results

http://www.estronaut.com/a/pap_smear_results_interpretation.htm

You get a Pap smear—now what do the results mean? This Estronaut site decodes the lab report. Read also **Taking Control of Your Pap Test** at http://www.estronaut.com/a/pap_test_control.htm.

Breast Exams

Combining monthly breast self-exams with yearly mammograms can help you catch breast cancer or other abnormalities early. The following sites tell you how and why to do a self-exam, and what to expect from a mammogram.

The Breast Self-Exam

http://breastdoctor.com/breast/exam.htm

You know you're supposed to do a breast self-exam monthly, but you're not sure how to do it. Get instructions from BreastDoctor.com. You can also learn about mammograms at http://breastdoctor.com/breast/mammogram/mammogram.htm.

Mammograms

http://www.wellweb.com/WOMEN/WMMAMMOG.HTM

Wellness Web describes what a mammogram is, how to choose a facility, what to expect, how to prepare, and how to follow up in this clear and comprehensive guide.

Mammography Links

http://www.stayhealthy.com/centers/women2.cfm?P=363

These mammography links from Stayhealthy.com include sites for information about breast health and breast cancer, not just mammograms.

Pregnancy

All of our Medical Super Sites and the content sites listed in this chapter have terrific pregnancy pages, with advice on everything from preconception to postpartum depression. In addition, check out the following pregnancy sites.

Healthy Pregnancy, Healthy Baby

http://www.fda.gov/fdac/features/1999/299_baby.html

Exercise, good food, and prenatal care are the keys to a healthy pregnancy. This *FDA Consumer* article gives advice about nutrition, medical care, and other lifestyle choices for a smooth pregnancy and healthy baby.

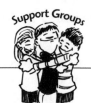

Support Groups

StorkSite

http://www.storksite.com

Are you pregnant or have you recently given birth? Become a "storkie" by joining this community of moms and moms-to-be that offers articles, shopping, chat, and message boards.

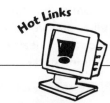

Hot Links

Exercise During Pregnancy

http://www.fitnesslink.com/women/pregnancy.shtml

Is exercise recommended during pregnancy? How much and what kind? This article from FitnessLink lists the reasons to exercise during pregnancy and offers guidelines from the American College of Obstetricians & Gynecologists.

Pregnancy Today

http://www.pregnancytoday.com

This site overflows with valuable information for moms-to-be and new mothers. Name your baby, develop your birth plan, read real-life birth stories, buy a good book, stay healthy throughout your pregnancy, or talk to others who have similar concerns.

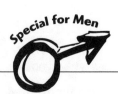

Dad, It's Your Baby, Too

http://www.healthystart.net/psa/man/dad_brochure.htm

This online brochure helps expectant dads deal with feelings, fears, and worries, as well as prepare for fatherhood while helping their partner have a healthy pregnancy and a healthy baby. This brochure is not very comprehensive, but it's a reassuring start.

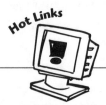

101 Reasons to Breastfeed Your Baby

http://www.promom.org/101/

Yep, 101 reasons—count 'em! Some are supported by scientific studies (such as "Formula feeding is associated with lower I.Q.") with the citations given; others are subjective (such as "Breastfed babies smell fantastic"), from ProMoM (Promotion of Mother's Milk, Inc.).

Childbirth.org

http://www.childbirth.org

"Birth is a natural process, not a medical procedure." What's a doula, and do you need one? Should you get an epidural? Can you have a VBAC? This site is an exhaustive resource for all your pregnancy and childbirth questions.

Pregnancy at About.com

http://pregnancy.about.com/

This quality site from About.com offers a multitude of pregnancy-related links, useful articles, due date forums, and a gallery of ultrasound photos!

BabyData.com

http://www.babydata.com/

"The premier website for pregnant couples and those trying to conceive" offers help in getting pregnant and tips on bringing a healthy child into the world. This renowned resource from Dr. Amos Grunebaum has been acquired by OnHealth.

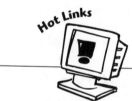

Circumcision: A Closer Look

http://www.healthcentral.com/specials/circumcision/
circumcision_intro.cfm

The American Academy of Pediatrics no longer routinely recommends circumcision for newborn males. Get Dean Edell's take on this controversial subject with this guide to male circumcision, including a description of circumcision surgery and photos of intact adult males.

Pregnancy & Baby's First Year

http://www.mayohealth.org/mayo/common/htm/baby_pg1.htm

Adapted from the Mayo Clinic's *Complete Book of Pregnancy & Baby's First Year*, this comprehensive site offers a wealth of information, organized by trimester or subject for easy access to exactly the topics you want.

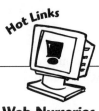

Web Nurseries

Awwww, this is so cute! Some hospitals are posting photos of newborns at their Web sites. If you have a baby there, you can email the URL of your baby photo instead of mailing actual photos to all your relatives. Take a look:

➤ http://www.bidmc.harvard.edu/baby/ Beth Israel Deaconess Medical Center, Boston, Massachusetts.

➤ http://www.bornatusa.com/ USA Children's & Women's Hospital, Mobile, Alabama.

➤ http://209.184.145.200/mcd/ Medical City Dallas Hospital, Dallas, Texas.

➤ http://www.webnursery.com/ First Foto is the company that produces the Web Nurseries. This site links you to all the hospitals that offer this program.

Infertility

Ten to fifteen percent of couples are affected by infertility, according to the Mayo Clinic. Infertility is defined as the inability to become pregnant after one year of frequent, unprotected sexual intercourse. This is different than sterility, which is the inability to conceive a child under any circumstance.

If you've been diagnosed as infertile, don't lose heart. This might simply mean that becoming pregnant will be a challenge. Medical treatments for infertility are close to amazing, so don't give up before thoroughly exploring your options. The following sites can help.

Overcoming Infertility

http://www.fda.gov/fdac/features/1997/197_fert.html

This article from *FDA Consumer* is an overview of infertility: causes, tests, and treatments. This is a good starting place for the basic information.

Fertile Thoughts

http://www.fertilethoughts.com/infertility/index.html

"A web community devoted to the needs of infertile couples and couples seeking to build a family through medical treatment of infertility." This site has everything: a complete online book on infertility (*Getting Pregnant: A Guide for the Infertile Couple* by Aniruddha Malpani, M.D., and his wife, Anjali Malpani, M.D.), chats, bulletin boards, personal histories, and links.

Atlanta Reproductive Health Centre WWW

http://www.ivf.com/

"Your infertility home on the Net" offers articles, videos, and an online book: *Miracle Babies and Other Happy Endings for Couples with Fertility Problems* by Mark Perloe, M.D., and Linda Gail Christie.

Infertility Center

http://www.womens-health.com/
health_center/infertility/index.html

This comprehensive learning center from Women's Health Interactive aims to empower couples who are dealing with infertility and their feelings and frustrations. You find extensive information here by clicking the different modules and the options on the navigation bar.

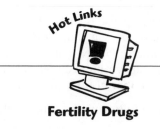

Fertility Drugs

http://www.mayohealth.org/
mayo/9902/htm/fertility.htm

This article from the Mayo Clinic describes seven fertility drugs, who should use them, how they work, and the course of treatment, plus questions to ask when deciding on a fertility drug.

INCIID

http://www.inciid.org/

The InterNational Council for Infertility Information Dissemination is "dedicated to helping infertile couples explore their family-building options, including treatment, adoption and choosing to live childfree." INCIID (pronounced "inside") offers dozens of fact sheets, plus bulletin boards (answered by experts) and chat rooms.

RESOLVE

http://www.resolve.org/

RESOLVE, the National Infertility Association, aims to provide "timely, compassionate support and information to individuals who are experiencing infertility issues." This site tells you where to start to determine if you have an infertility problem and how to choose an infertility specialist. RESOLVE also connects you to other people with the same concerns through live local chapters.

Menopause

A generation ago, women didn't talk about menopause. We're talking up a storm now. At parties, in gym locker rooms, at coffee breaks, and now online, we're discussing hot flashes, urine leaks, and vaginal dryness with as little embarrassment as we once compared diets, men, or child-rearing techniques. We're hungry for information, and we're eager to share what we're learning and our opinions about our options.

Menopause is such a huge concern that it should have its own chapter. In fact, it *did* have its own chapter (Chapter 23) in *The Complete Idiot's Guide to Online Health and Fitness*. You're invited to use that power-surging energy to explore all the information about symptoms, medical and alternative treatments, support, and marvelous sites that Shannon Entin and I found for you in that book.

The following are some highlights.

FAQs About Menopause

http://www.menopause.org/aboutm/faq.html

This site has an excellent Frequently Asked Questions section about menopause that covers not only the basics, but also detailed information about phytoestrogens (foods that contain estrogen-like properties) and different therapies.

Discovery Health

http://www.discoveryhealth.com

Click **Her Health**, **Woman and Aging**, **Menopause** to find a variety of articles on menopause basics, symptoms, HRT, natural therapies, and related conditions. The material is provided by Johns Hopkins, the National Institutes of Health (NIH), and other reputable sources.

Menopause Guidebook

http://www.menopause.org/mgintro.htm

This online booklet from the North American Menopause Society helps you "make informed Healthcare decisions at midlife." The content is extensive and conservative, pointing out where more research is needed to determine the value of particular therapies.

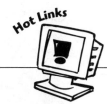

Self-Care Advisor: Menopause

http://my.webmd.com/self_care_article/DMK_ARTICLE_58325

This helpful article describes the symptoms of menopause, and what to do about them. Learn self-care procedures for relieving hot flashes, night sweats, vaginal dryness, and emotional stress—plus advice for when to see a doctor.

Menopause

http://www.nih.gov/health/chip/nia/menop/men1.htm

This site from the National Institute of Aging explains the basics: What menopause is (the rather dry explanation spiced up with quotes from and photos of real women), what to expect, long-term effects, and hormone replacement therapy (an unbiased report of the benefits and risks, with a pro/con chart).

Doctor's Guide to Menopause Information & Resources

http://www.pslgroup.com/Menopause.htm

This site's mission is to provide "the information and information services most likely to help promote the informed and appropriate use of medicines by health care professionals and organizations as well as by the people to whom they are prescribed." You'll find "medical news and alerts" summarizing research in menopause medications, basic information about menopause and HRT, discussion groups, newsgroups, and links.

Menopause Resource Guide

http://www.4woman.org/owh/pub/menoguide.htm

The National Women's Health Information Center, from the U.S. Public Health Service's Office on Women's Health, Department of Health and Human Services, provides this guide, with many links and lists, including dozens of helpful books.

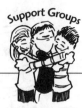

Menopause Support Groups

Nobody understands what a menopausal woman is experiencing like another sleep-deprived, irritable, hot-flashing woman, and plenty are online ready to gripe, laugh, moan, and exchange stories.

➤ Visit the Hot Flash site at `http://www.families-first.com/hotflash/`, and then subscribe to its mailing list at `http://www.onelist.com/subscribe.cgi/hotflash`.

➤ Add yourself to the "Menopaus" mailing list at `http://www.howdyneighbor.com/menopaus/listinfo.htm`.

➤ Visit the Power Surge chats and bulletin boards at `http://www.dearest.com`.

➤ Participate in a menopause newsgroup at `alt.support.menopause`.

Preventing Violence

Violence against women has come out of the closet to some extent, but public awareness hasn't solved the problem. Consider these statistics from the Society for Women's Health Research (`http://www.womens-health.org/factsheet.html#violence`) and the Family Violence Prevention Fund (`http://www.fvpf.org/facts/`):

➤ Thirty-one percent of women in the United States are physically or sexually abused by a husband or boyfriend at some point in their lives.

➤ Twenty percent of women's visits to emergency rooms are due to battering.

➤ Fifty percent of men who assault their wives also abuse their children.

➤ Ninety percent of women who have been physically abused by their partners do not discuss these incidents with their physicians.

➤ Fifty-seven percent of women who have been physically abused by their partners do not discuss the incidents with anyone.

If you're in an abusive situation, realize that help exists, and that you've got to get out. The following sites will give you the knowledge and support to help you take the first steps away from your abuser.

Getting Help

http://www.fvpf.org/gethelp/index.html

Are you ever afraid of your partner? Has your partner threatened to harm you? This site assures you that you are not alone, and advises you what to do, including devising a personal safety plan and a workplace safety plan.

Jane Doe Inc.

http://www.besafe.org/

This helpful guide takes you through the steps of figuring out if you need help from domestic violence and learning how to get it. This guide also addresses same-sex domestic-violence issues. Jane Doe Inc. is the Massachusetts Coalition Against Sexual Assault and Domestic Violence.

Commission on Domestic Violence

http://www.abanet.org/domviol/home.html

This site from the American Bar Association's Commission on Domestic Violence presents a self-test to see if you are a victim of spousal or partner abuse, gives you phone numbers for getting help, and offers help for getting legal aid, even if you can't afford a lawyer.

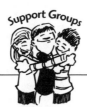

Support Groups

Women Online Worldwide

http://www.wowwomen.com/

Click **Message Boards, Guest Access** (to take a look before registering), **Women Online Worldwide, Violence Against Women**. You'll read women's stories about their abuse and plenty of supportive responses.

The Least You Need to Know

➤ You can find information and support about any women's health issue online.

➤ If you're pregnant, infertile, or menopausal, you can find extensive information and wisdom from experts and from other women going through the same circumstance.

➤ You can educate yourself about women's screening tests so that you know what to expect.

➤ If you're a victim of abuse, learn about safety measures to protect yourself, and then get help and get out.

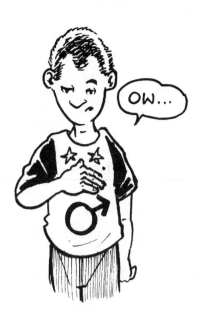

Chapter 9

Men's Health

In This Chapter

➤ The importance of regular check-ups

➤ How to keep your prostate healthy

➤ Cautions for ordering impotence treatments online

➤ Facts about hair-loss treatments

Are you a man who is feeling a bit short-changed surfing the Web for information about male health topics? Does it seem as though many health sites are geared more toward women's concerns? You're not imagining things. In truth, women make an estimated 80 percent of health-care decisions and almost 60 percent of health-care purchases, according to a 1999 Jupiter Analyst Report. Some health sites report that more than 75 percent of their visitors are women. So you can see why the Web-content decision makers and advertisers are targeting women.

But you're a decisive guy, and you want to get a handle on your health concerns. This chapter shows you where you can find information about the topics that are most requested by men, and where you can explore other issues that interest you.

If you don't find the topic you're looking for here, look in Chapter 20, "Cancer," (for testicular cancer, for example) and in Chapter 10, "Sexuality" (for vasectomy, for example).

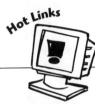

Hot Links

Suggested Guidelines for Regular Examinations and Preventive Measures for Men

http://www.malehealthcenter.com/Selfcare.html#anchor20210916

How often should you have a physical exam? A rectal exam? A tetanus shot? Find out from this list of exams and preventive treatments.

Getting a Checkup

I know, I know—real men don't like to go to doctors. Doctors do weird things with gloved fingers and ask embarrassing questions. Unfortunately, though, real men who don't go to doctors cheat themselves out of the likelihood of detecting a life-threatening disease early enough for the best management or a cure. In my opinion, real men ask directions—directions about maintaining a healthy body, that is. And the person who can give personalized directions for you is your personal physician.

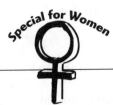

Special for Women

What Can a Woman Do for a Man's Health?

http://www.malehealthcenter.com/Woman.html#anchor573831

This article from the Male Health Center is directed at women. Learn how and why the way to a man's health is through a woman, and 15 things a woman can do to keep a man healthy.

If you think I'm ragging on you unnecessarily, check out the following stats:

➤ One-third of American men have not had a checkup in the past year.

➤ Nine million men haven't seen a doctor in five years.

➤ Men have 150 million fewer doctor visits than women every year, across all age groups.

➤ Men under 65 have 2.5 times more heart attacks than women; yet women are more likely than men to get their blood pressure checked.

➤ Men are at greater risk of stress-related illnesses than women, yet women comprise 80 percent of the participants in stress-management programs.

➤ More than 3 million men have early Type 2 diabetes and don't know it.

Read these and more scary statistics that should send you marching to your physician's office in *Why Men Don't Go to the Doctor*, from the Male Health Center (http://www.malehealthcenter.com/Bullet.html#anchor137891).

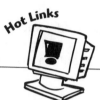

Hot Links

How to Choose (and Get Maximum Mileage from) Your Primary Care Doctor

http://www.coolware.com/health/medical_reporter/choosing.html

"More often than not, we end up in a doctor's office only because we were forced to, by a cold that wouldn't quit, a stomach pain that became unbearable, or a sore knee that threatened our ski getaway. For some of us, a check-up happens only by ultimatum from one's employer. In fact, it's possible your car gets better care than you do." This article from *Rose Men's Health Resource* in Denver uses a breezy style to give important information: the need for a primary care physician, how to choose one, questions to ask when you're prospecting for one, and how to get the most out of your doctor.

Prostate Health

The prostate is the gland about the size of a walnut surrounding the urethra and immediately below the bladder in males. Don't mispronounce it as *prostrate*, which means lying down flat on the ground.

As men age, it is essential to examine the prostate. Half of men over 50 and up to 90 percent of men over age 80 have a non-cancerous condition known as benign prostatic hyperplasia (BPH), which is an enlargement of the prostate that leads to difficulty urinating. More distressing, prostate cancer is the number one cancer for men, affecting almost all men by the time they reach the age of 80. (Lung cancer affects slightly fewer men, but causes four times as many deaths.)

Sixty-three percent of men diagnosed with prostate cancer will survive at least 10 years and 89 percent will survive at least five years, according to the American Cancer Society. These survival rates are partly due to improved screening tests and diagnostics that discover cancer in early stages. (Read more in Chapter 20.) All the more reason to bite the bullet and insert that finger.

Getting the Exam

Far more men would detect prostate disease early enough to treat it successfully if they requested both the digital rectal exam and the prostate-specific antigen blood test from their doctors.

The prostate is right below the bladder and in front of the rectum, and it's easy for a doctor to examine it by inserting a rubber-gloved finger into the rectum. This might not be your idea of a good time, but it's easy, and your doc knows how to make it painless.

Examining Yourself

Between doctor's appointments, it's important to examine your own prostate. The following site shows you how.

The Prostate Self Exam

`http://www.healthcentral.com/specials/prostate_exam.cfm`

Dr. Dean Edell explains exactly how to do a prostate self-exam or teach your partner to do it.

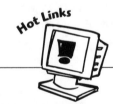

Hot Links

Impotence Resource Site

`http://www.impotence.org/`

The American Foundation for Urologic Disease invites you to learn more about what is often called "the most common untreated, treatable medical disorder in the United States." Read articles about impotence, including causes, treatments, and the importance of talking to your partner and your doctor about it.

Erectile Dysfunction

Erectile dysfunction is a fancy word for impotence, the inability to achieve or sustain an erection. Eighty percent of impotence has physical causes. Nearly 95 percent of all cases can be successfully treated after the cause is determined.

Knowing the cause is essential. Erectile dysfunction can be a symptom of another medical disorder that needs prompt attention, such as heart disease, cancer, or diabetes. Do not delay a possible life-saving diagnosis by bypassing the urologic work-up.

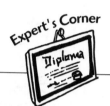

Facts About Impotence

Perhaps the most difficult part of impotence involves separating fact from fiction. These facts from the American Foundation for Urologic Disease will help you understand impotence better:

➤ Impotence is NOT "all in your head." Approximately 20 percent of impotence can be attributed to psychological causes. It is usually a secondary condition brought on by other physical causes. In fact, evaluation by a physician might save your life!

➤ Erectile difficulty is frequently the first sign of vascular disease, which could lead to a heart attack or stroke. It might also be a first sign of diabetes.

➤ Impotence is usually NOT a normal consequence of aging. It's true that the likelihood of impotence increases as you get older, but erectile difficulty is more likely the result of medical problems that occur at a greater rate as a man ages.

➤ Impotence is NOT just a man's problem. Because it can disrupt marriages, relationships, and the way sufferers feel about themselves, impotence is a couple's problem. In fact, treatment success rates are even higher when both partners are involved.

➤ Impotence is NOT permanent! About 95 percent of all impotence can be successfully treated after the cause has been determined.

—From *Impotence Resource Site* by the American Foundation for Urologic Disease, http://www.impotence.org/facts

Viagra

The best known treatment for erectile dysfunction is that miracle drug, Viagra. But be careful. The truth is that you can go online, do a search for the keyword Viagra, and have a gang of sites battling for a chance to fill your order. You don't have a prescription? No problem—just fill out a questionnaire, and you're approved for the drug, even if you fill in your cat's name (Pretty Kitty), age, and weight. This isn't healthy, guys, especially if you have an underlying condition that isn't getting diagnosed. And Viagra isn't the right drug for men taking nitrates for a heart condition.

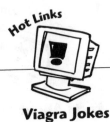

Viagra Jokes

http://www.net2business.com/humor/viagra.html

"Have you tried the new hot beverage, Viagraccino? One cup and you're up all night." If you need a quick Viagra joke to share with the guys (or gals), you can find it here.

Fake Viagra

You're surfing along, and you come upon a "natural" cure for impotence. Watch out. If the product being pitched to cure impotence is "herbal" or "all natural," forget it. So far, no "herbal" or "all natural" substance has been shown to be an effective treatment for impotence.

Also be cautious when you come across a drug with a brand name that is sort of spelled like Viagra but not quite. Can you spell C-O-N? The intent is to confuse you so you think you're ordering the real thing. You're not.

This is the bottom line: Check out any treatment with your doctor first.

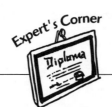

Expert's Corner

See Your Doc

"If you are having an erectile problem, you need to see a doctor and get a check-up, not order Viagra or a Viagra substitute online. Of 207 men who went to a urology clinic for treatment of erectile dysfunction, 15 percent of them had cancer—prostate, bladder, kidney, or penile cancer. Impotence can also indicate heart disease, or diabetes. So, please, friends, if you value your health, don't rely on an online pharmacy or an over-the-counter "remedy" for erectile dysfunction. That online doctor can't give you an exam—and that herbal supplement maker won't get a medical history before you buy that pill."

—Dean Edell, M.D., `http://www.healthcentral.com`

Virility Plus

Admit it, in the depths of your soul, don't you wish you could anonymously order a safe, less-expensive Viagra substitute without the hassle of a prescription or an awkward doctor's visit, and enjoy erections at will? Type in the following URL for Virility Plus.

Virility Plus

`www.ari.net/virilityplus`

"Say farewell to impotence!" screams the headline. "The American Academy of Urology introduces Virility Plus® the safe and all natural alternative to Viagra!" (See Figure 9.1.) Goodness sakes, that sounds credible, doesn't it? The American Academy of Urology wouldn't back anything shady. (If you've taken our PILOT method to heart, I'm asking you to suspend your well-founded skepticism for a few minutes.)

And the price, $69.95 for a 3-month supply, is certainly cheaper than Viagra's $10 a pill (as long as you're planning to have sex more than 2.3 times a month), and—now this is cool—you don't even need a prescription!

Is your scam meter going crazy? Keep reading.

The ad goes on to say that Virility Plus® is available exclusively from the American Academy of Urology, "the nation's leading scientific research organization devoted to male sexual dysfunction."

Figure 9.1

Virility Plus entices you with an alluring claim.

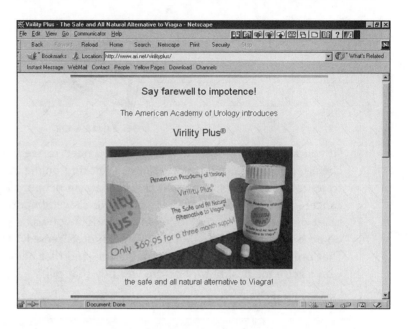

Next we get a description of the "ancient Scandinavian formula" on which Virility Plus® is based, with "the curative powers of Yohimbe, once used by the Vikings to boost male sexual potency." Vikings—now those were virile men!

Keep scrolling to read about the "double-blind, placebo-controlled clinical trials"—no journal references, but what the heck—that scientifically prove that Virility Plus can "reverse impotence in clinically diagnosed impotent men…even those who have been unable to have sexual intercourse for more than five years."

A "scientific" explanation of how the product works follows, from "Dr. Bjorn Bergmann, renowned Swedish physician," who concludes, "Virility Plus® consistently performed better than Viagra without the risks and side-effects." Gosh, why haven't we ever heard of this when we've all heard of Viagra? Must be the pharmaceutical industry conspiracy.

I really like the part that says, "No Embarassing Doctor Visits!" Yes, "embarrassing" is misspelled!

If you're following along on the Web site, click **Order Now!**.

Here's where you discover that you've been reading a fake ad for a fake Viagra from the real Federal Trade Commission (FTC), posted "to spotlight the hazards of impotence treatment scams marketed on the Internet"!

You could have figured out yourself that this product had to be bogus. The "American Academy of Urology" doesn't exist, and if it did, and if it were the research organization it claims to be, it would not be retailing the product it just impartially tested. Duhhh. Besides, after you run the PILOT method on this site, you see every red flag wave wildly at you.

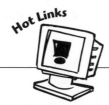

Hot Links

The Truth About Impotence Treatment Claims

http://www.ftc.gov/bcp/conline/pubs/alerts/impoalrt.htm

"Recent advances in treating impotence have opened the floodgates for bogus remedies for this condition." The Federal Trade Commission offers tips for evaluating claims you might want to believe, but shouldn't.

Hair Today, Gone Tomorrow

In 1150 B.C., Egyptians covered their baldness with a mixture of fats from ibex (a mountain goat), lion, crocodile, serpent, goose, and hippopotamus. Both Julius Caesar and Napoleon grew their hair long in the back and combed it forward over their bald spots. Age, hormones, and genetics combine to create the male pattern hair loss that has plagued men for centuries.

Minoxidil (marketed as Rogaine or as generic minoxidil, which is just as effective as the brand name, and less expensive) and finasteride (marketed as Propecia) are the only FDA-approved treatments for hair loss. Hair additions and hair-replacement surgery are more natural-looking than they used to be, and these might be another solution.

The following sites educate you about male-pattern hair loss and describe methods for treating or coping with it.

Hair Replacement: What Works, What Doesn't

http://www.fda.gov/fdac/features/1997/397_hair.html

Combating and covering up hair loss has become an estimated $1-billion-a-year industry. This fact-filled article from the FDA describes minoxidil (it was written before finasteride was approved), surgical procedures, hairpieces, and cosmetics, and warns you against fraudulent treatments.

Baldness Treatments

http://mayohealth.org/mayo/9607/htm/hair_rep.htm

The Mayo Clinic debunks hair-growth schemes that you find on the Web and on late-night television, then discusses the merits of minoxodil, finasteride, and surgery.

American Hair Loss Council Online Brochures

`http://www.ahlc.org/info.html`

Read online brochures from the American Hair Loss Council on hair replacement surgery, non-surgical hair additions, male pattern hair loss, and other topics.

Start Here: Men's Health Sites

Learn about a variety of men's health topics from the following sites, hand-picked to make your searching easier.

Not for Men Only: The Male Health Center

`http://www.malehealthcenter.com/`

"Treating the whole man, not just parts," this men's health site is from the Male Health Center in Dallas, Texas, with articles on every aspect of men's health: symptoms, self-care, food, exercise, and erections (see Figure 9.2). Check out the "His Health" columns by Dr. Ken Goldberg that cover nearly every subject that concerns men.

Figure 9.2

The Male Health Center is a gold mine of men's health information.

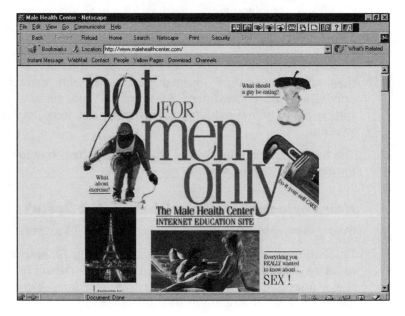

Men's Health

`http://www1.sympatico.ca/healthyway/COMMUNITIES/men_com.html`

This site from Healthy Way offers articles and news on an assortment of health-related topics of special interest to men: Peyronie's disease, safe shaving, golf swings, and vasectomies, for example.

Men's Health Center

`http://www.mayohealth.org/mayo/common/htm/menspg2.htm`

The Mayo Clinic's men's site has links to a variety of articles on appearance, prostate and testicular cancer, urologic conditions, reproduction, and sexuality, plus breaking news about men's health topics.

Men's Health in Conditions A–Z

`http://onhealth.com/ch1/resource/conditions/sub6.asp`

This site from OnHealth covers male health topics such as heart disease, prostate health, impotence, balanitis (penile yeast infection), cryptorchidism (undescended testicle), jock itch, hair loss, and every STD known to man.

Just for You: Men

`http://www.healthfinder.com/justforyou/men/Default.htm`

This men's health information page from HealthFinder offers reviewed links to informational sites about physical activity, impotence, prostate problems, sports medicine, STD prevention, tobacco information, contraception, Viagra, and more.

Ask NOAH About: Men's Health

`http://www.noah.cuny.edu/healthyliving/menshealth.html`

This site from New York Online Access to Health (NOAH) has many reviewed links to sites on all the men's health topics you hope to find, including fatherhood, male fertility, plastic surgery for men, and primary care for men.

Men's Health Zone

`http://www.intelihealth.com/` (click Men's Health)

This men's site from InteliHealth presents information from Johns Hopkins on prostate cancer, cholesterol, heart disease, impotence, hair loss, fitness and exercise, aging, and being a new father (see Figure 9.3).

Figure 9.3

InteliHealth from Johns Hopkins offers reliable and interesting information about men's health.

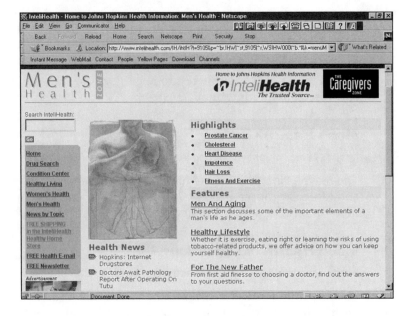

The Least You Need to Know

➤ It's essential to see your physician regularly; surfing the Web for medical information just isn't enough.

➤ You can (and should) examine your own prostate, as well as make regular appointments for a prostate exam.

➤ Do not treat erectile dysfunction without getting a medical diagnosis, and beware of ordering impotence treatments online.

➤ You can learn about hair-loss treatments online.

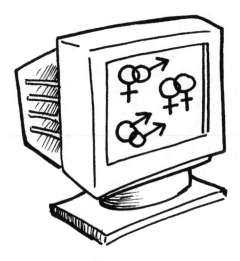

Chapter 10

Sexuality

In This Chapter

➤ Getting facts about sex and sexual health online

➤ Finding non-judgmental information about sexual orientation

➤ Evaluating which birth control method is for you, with online help

➤ Learning about sexually transmitted diseases and how to prevent them

➤ Finding sex therapy online

This chapter shows you how to use the Internet to find information that answers some of your health questions about sexuality. The Web is a superb resource, whether you want to learn about birth control, sexual orientation, STDs, or a way to explain the birds and the bees to your child. For information about impotence (erectile dysfunction), refer to Chapter 9, "Men's Health." For information about infertility and pregnancy, refer to Chapter 8, "Women's Health."

This is a health book, realize, so you won't find porn sites in this chapter. (If you're interested in exploring, uh, other areas of Internet sexuality, *The Complete Idiot's Guide to Sex on the Net* might be your ticket to titillation.)

The Birds, the Bees, and the Web: Learning About Sexuality

The Web eliminates those embarrassing forays into library stacks to learn about your own or the other gender's reproductive system and sexual responses. Although talking to your doctor is always recommended, you no longer have to get up the nerve to ask your physician whether a particular desire or response is normal. The Web might even cut down on the whispered misinformation passed between preteens if they knew where to find sites like the ones in this chapter. The following sites explain sex frankly, non-judgmentally, and without making a big deal of it.

Sexuality

http://sexuality.about.com/

Learn about female condoms, sexual dysfunction, the contraceptive sponge, and the "dildo laws" in Georgia. This site from About.com includes informative articles about and helpful links to all different topics of sexual health.

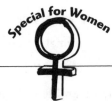

A Woman's Guide to Sexuality

http://www.plannedparenthood.org/WOMENSHEALTH/sexuality.htm

This guide from Planned Parenthood is intended to help women of all ages make informed decisions about their sex lives. It gives an overview of the decisions, thoughts, and feelings that women experience about their sexuality.

Sexuality Bytes

http://www.sexualitybytes.ninemsn.com.au/adult/

"Come inside and find all the ingredients for a healthy sex life, with info and photos on hundreds of topics from petting and foreplay to childbirth to growing old, and everything in between." This Australian site is an online encyclopedia of sex and sexual health.

The Sexual Health Infocenter

http://www.sexhealth.org/infocenter/

This site offers overviews to better sex, sex and aging, safer sex, sexual problems, STDs, and lesbian/gay issues. Though it doesn't go very deeply into these topics, it's a good place to start.

Sexual Health Network

http://www.sexualhealth.com/

People with disabilities or other health problems might experience sexual difficulties. "Sexual Health Network is dedicated to providing easy access to sexuality information, education, counseling, therapy, medical attention, and other sexuality resources for people with disability, illness, or other health related problems."

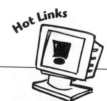

Hot Links

Everything You Ever Wanted to Know About the G-Spot

http://www.minou.com/aboutsex/gspot.htm

Where is that dang G-spot? This site shows you where it is, how you can find it, and sure-to-please methods for stimulating it.

Discussing Birds and Bees

http://www.mayohealth.org/mayo/9909/htm/kids.htm

How do you cope with children's sexual questions and behavior? First take a deep breath, then read this article from the Mayo Clinic about sexuality in your preschool child, early school-age child, and teenager.

Go Ask Alice

http://www.goaskalice.columbia.edu/

This popular, controversial site from Columbia University's Health Education Program is accessed more than 2.5 million times a month, mostly by high school and college students. It aims "to provide factual, in-depth, straight-forward, and nonjudgmental information to assist readers' decision-making about their physical, sexual, emotional, and spiritual health." "Alice" answers explicit questions about relationships and sexuality and offers 1,600 previously posted questions and answers.

Iwannaknow.org

`http://www.iwannaknow.org/`

Should I have sex? Can I get a STD from a tattoo parlor? This teen-friendly site provides answers to questions about teen sexual health and STDs from the American Social Health Association, which is dedicated to increasing awareness of sexually transmitted diseases.

SIECUS Parent's Area

`http://www.siecus.org/parent/pare0000.html`

SIECUS (Sex Information and Education Council of the United States) helps you educate your children about sexuality with articles like "Communication Tips for Parents" and "Kids Online: What Parents Can Do to Protect Their Children From Cyberspace."

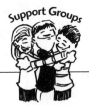

Support Groups

Support Links Page

`http://www.sfsi.org/links/support.html`

San Francisco Sex Information is a free information and referral switchboard providing anonymous, accurate, non-judgmental information about sex by telephone (415-989-SFSI, Monday through Friday from 3 P.M. to 9 P.M. Pacific time). This site presents links to support for an abundance of sex issues and sexual orientations, such as sex workers, gays and lesbians (and their parents, ex-spouses, and so on), teens, teen parents, victims of sexual assault, people with herpes, and more.

Sexual Orientation

Human sexuality is complex and doesn't fit into neat, orderly categories or labels. Some people are attracted to the other gender, some to the same gender, and some to both genders. Even within one predominant orientation, there is a "sliding scale" of attraction, curiosity, and desire for relationship. We're all different.

Teenagers who find themselves attracted to the same gender often feel like misfits. They might be treated like outcasts by their peers, who are trying to come to terms with their own sexuality, and this sometimes takes the form of ostracizing and taunting those who are different. They are often lonely, lack role models, and fear confiding in adults or other teens.

The Web comes to the rescue by offering non-judgmental, informative, and affirming sites for all sexual orientations.

!OutProud! Brochures

http://www.outproud.org/brochures.html

These online brochures are aimed at youth who are "gay, lesbian, bisexual, still figuring things out, or someone who just wants to better understand what it means to be a lesbigay individual." Topics include being yourself, how to come out to your parents, and watching out for yourself in online relationships.

PFLAG

http://pflag.org/pflag.html

Parents, Families, and Friends of Lesbians and Gays (PFLAG) "provides opportunity for dialogue about sexual orientation and gender identity, and acts to create a society that is healthy and respectful of human diversity." Click **resources** to read online booklets and links.

Gay and Lesbian Adolescents

http://www.aacap.org/publications/factsfam/63.htm

This article from the American Academy of Child & Adolescent Psychiatry reassures parents that homosexual orientation is not a mental disorder and helps them understand their gay teenagers' isolation, worries, and fears.

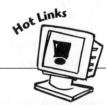

Hot Links

Answers to Your Questions About Sexual Orientation and Homosexuality

http://pflag.org/store/resource/apa.html

This article from the American Psychological Association discusses what causes a person to have a particular sexual orientation, that homosexuality isn't a mental illness, and why therapy to "change" sexual orientation is unnecessary and may be harmful.

Birth Control

If you want to avoid pregnancy, the Web offers plenty of resources to compare methods and reach the decision that is best for you and your partner.

Contraception

The Web offers plenty of information about contraception methods. Most of our Medical Super Sites can be good introductions, or start with the following sites.

Protecting Against Unintended Pregnancy: A Guide to Contraceptive Choices

http://www.fda.gov/fdac/features/1997/397_baby.html

This article from *FDA Consumer* describes the FDA-approved methods of birth control, including barrier methods, spermicides, hormonal methods, and IUDs.

Planned Parenthood

http://www.plannedparenthood.org/

Learn about birth control, emergency contraception, abortion, STDs, reproductive rights, and more.

Voluntary Sterilization

If you're sure you don't want to have children (or more children), you'll have fewer worries about birth control if you get a tubal ligation if you're a woman or a vasectomy if you're a man. The following sites tell you more about these procedures.

Voluntary Sterilization

http://www.noah.cuny.edu/sexuality/ushc/vsterilization.html

Learn the facts about vasectomy and tubal ligation in simple, reassuring language from NOAH.

All About Vasectomy

http://www.plannedparenthood.org/BIRTH-CONTROL/allaboutvas.htm

Planned Parenthood explains how vasectomy works and its low risks, and answers all your questions in simple, direct language.

Sexually Transmitted Diseases

STD means sexually transmitted disease, also known as venereal disease. This broad term refers to more than 50 diseases and syndromes that may be transmitted sexually, usually through the exchange of body fluids, such as semen, vaginal secretions, and blood.

According to the American Social Health Association:

➤ One in five people in the United States has an STD.

➤ Two-thirds of all STDs occur in people 25 years of age or younger.

➤ One in four new STD infections occur in teenagers.

Identifying STDs is easier with the help of the Web, but please don't self-diagnose. See a physician immediately if you have any of the symptoms described or pictured in the following sites.

Sexually Transmitted Diseases

http://healthydevil.stuaff.duke.edu

Click **sexually transmitted diseases (STDs)** to learn about the causes, symptoms, treatments, and risks of not treating STDs such as chlamydia, crabs, gonorrhea, herpes, and syphilis from Healthy Devil Online, from the Health Education staff and health-care providers at Duke University (see Figure 10.1).

Figure 10.1

Healthy Devil Online tells you how to recognize symptoms of a variety of STDs.

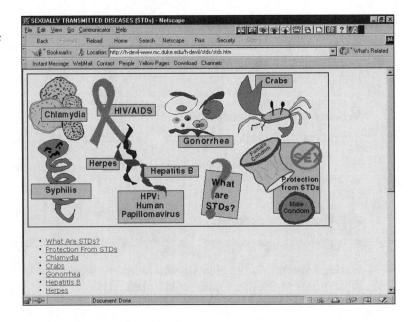

What Do the Symptoms of STDs Look Like?

http://www.thebody.com/sowadsky/symptoms/symptoms.html

View close-up, color photos of what syphilis, gonorrhea, chlamydia, genital warts, and other STDs look like on a penis, vulva, or anus. This site by Rick Sowadsky, MSPH, Nevada AIDS Hotline Coordinator, is not for the squeamish.

Safer Sex

You've heard the terms "safe sex" and "safer sex" bandied about. If neither you nor your partner has any STD, and you are in a committed, long-term, monogamous relationship, you don't have to worry about STD risk. For everyone else, sex is a gamble with any exchange of body fluids (blood, semen, vaginal secretions). "Safer sex" uses barriers like condoms and dental dams so that body fluids don't mix, minimizing the risk of disease transmission. The following sites teach you more about safer sex.

Guide to Safer Sex (Concise)

http://www.sexuality.org/concise.html

This brief, frank discussion of safer sex from the Society of Human Sexuality focuses on the basics of safer sex and how to make the precautions you choose feel as pleasurable as possible. If you want more, read the longer "Guide to Safer Sex (Lengthy)" at http://www.sexuality.org/safesex.html.

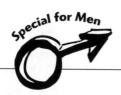

Condoms: A User's Guide

`http://www.mayohealth.org/mayo/9702/htm/condom_g.htm`

This article from the Mayo Clinic gives you straightforward pointers about how to choose and use a condom.

Condomania

`http://www.condomania.com/safer.sex`

"The Chinese made condoms out of oiled silk paper, Europeans used fish bladder, and Egyptians used papyrus soaked in water." Learn what's new in condom technology and design from this shopping site for condoms, with entertaining information you won't read anywhere else. Read condom reviews from popular magazines. Use the "Condom Wizard" to select your best brand and style. Click **safer sex**, then **educational information**, and then **manual** to read a safer-sex online booklet.

Safersex.Org

`http://www.safersex.org/safer.sex`

This site published by the Bisexual Resource Center presents frank, explicit articles about the risks of various types of sexual activity, how to put on a condom, and even gives tips on how to talk to a partner about "smart sex."

When Sex Is a Compulsion

If you or a loved one has a problem with sex being obsessive, self-destructive, or destructive to others, using the Internet for information can be an important first step to getting help. Use the following sites for learning and guidance, but please also seek professional help.

National Council on Sexual Addiction and Compulsivity

`http://www.ncsac.org/`

Read articles book recommendations on sex addiction and sexual offending (engaging in illegal sexual behaviors which involve victimization).

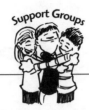

12-Step Groups

`http://www.ncsac.org/twelve_step.htm`

This site from the National Council on Sexual Addiction and Compulsivity has a list of different 12-step support groups for sex addicts, their families, and victims of sexual trauma. Some have Web sites; others have addresses and phone numbers to get information about live meetings.

The Sexual Addiction Screening Test

`http://www.sexhelp.com/sast.cfm`

Patrick J. Carnes, Ph.D., noted sex addictionologist and author, offers three versions of a sexual addiction screening test that provides a profile of responses which help to discriminate between addictive and nonaddictive behaviors. See also Dr. Carnes's Web links page: `http://www.sexhelp.com/links.cfm`.

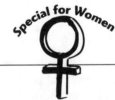

Women Sex Addicts

`http://www.ncsac.org/women_sex_addicts.htm`

This position paper from the National Council on Sexual Addiction and Compulsivity describes behaviors that indicate sexual addiction in women and suggests some ways to stop the behaviors, deal with the underlying feelings, and integrate healthy sexual behavior into their lives.

Expert's Corner

"Virtually everyone has the ability to choose how to express their sexual impulses. The concept of sexual addiction colludes with some people's desire to shirk responsibility for their sexual choices."

—Marty Klein, Ph.D., sex therapist, `http://www.sexed.org` (Read Dr. Klein's *Why There's No Such Thing as Sexual Addiction—And Why It really Matters* at `http://www.sexed.org/arch/arch08.htm` for more on this topic.)

Sex Therapy

Your need for information and assistance might go beyond reading articles. Some sites from sex therapists have Q&A or FAQ sections where you can read answers to sex questions. You can even pay a fee to have a sex therapist answer your very personal question. If you're struggling with a sexual problem, though, you can inform yourself online, but then get a live sex therapist or counselor who can guide you toward understanding and dealing with your issues.

Online

The following sites offer online answers to common and unique questions about sexual health, desire, behavior, and more.

Dr. Ruth

`http://www.drruth.com/`

Feisty sex therapist Dr. Ruth Westheimer presents Q&As, tips, and a message board, which might already have answers to your questions. You can even download sound clips of Dr. Ruth saying "Bravo!" or "You are a real smart cookie!" or an image of sperm meeting egg for your desktop background!

drDrew.Com

`http://www.DrDrew.com/`

Fans of Dr. Drew who appreciate his frank answers to sex questions on MTV's Loveline will be glad to know that he has a Web site. This site isn't just about sex. In fact, it welcomes all ages to forums and chats on a variety of health topics, with strict rules to protect the young, so you have to scout around a bit to find the sex talk.

(Hint: click **dr. drew's office**, and then look to the right under **frequently asked questions**, click **more topics at the arrow at the end of the list**, and aha!)

Sex Coach

`http://www.ivillage.com/relationships/archive/0,4142,101,00.html`

If you don't want to type in all those numbers, go to `http://www.ivillage.com/`, click **Relationships**, then look under Experts for **Sex Coach**. You find answers by Patti Britton, Ph.D., iVillage's Sex Coach, to more than 100 sex questions in categories such as Get the Facts on Sex, Improve Your Sex Life, Bedroom Crisis, Cybersex and Online Affairs, and Sex & Your Health.

Ask Me Anything

`http://www.SexEd.org/askme.htm`

Need a short answer to a big question? Read this archive of questions answered by sex therapist Marty Klein on topics as diverse as vaginal tightness, penile enlargement, trouble reaching orgasm, lack of desire, and infidelity.

Sex Therapy Online

`http://www.sexology.org/`

A sex therapist will answer one question or discuss one area of sexuality in a private email consultation for $75.

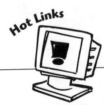

Hot Links

Finding a Sex Therapist

`http://sexuality.about.com/health/fitness/sexuality/library/weekly/aa062298.htm`

This article by Sandor Gardos, Ph.D., discusses how to choose a sex therapist. Click **article** by Robert Birch, Ph.D., when you get to that reference for a detailed article, *Your Introduction to Sex Therapy: What's It All About?*

Live

If you're looking for a real, live, face-to-face, local therapist to help you with a sexual issue, the following sites can help you find the right one.

American Association of Sex Educators, Counselors, and Therapists

`http://www.aasect.org/html/findatherapist.html`

Find a certified sex therapist or counselor in your geographic area. This referral service is still in the process of getting online, so if you don't find a therapist close enough, write for more referrals.

Look Up a Therapist

`http://www.sexologist.org/map/referral.htm`

Find a sex therapist in your area who is certified by the American Board of Sexology, and read about his or her specialties.

The Least You Need to Know

➤ You can find health-oriented information about sex, birth control, and STDs online.

➤ Teens can learn about sexual orientation and the facts of life from informative, non-judgmental, non-exploitative Web sites from credible sources.

➤ Sex therapists will answer questions online, but if you have a sexual issue that is interfering with your life, see a local sex therapist.

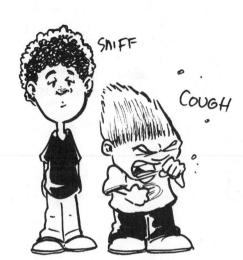

Chapter 11

Children's Health

In This Chapter

➤ Finding answers online to questions about your child's health

➤ Using the Internet for advice, support, research, and education about your child's illness

➤ Using the Web to educate your children on healthy habits

Searches for children's health information make up about 15 percent of health searches on the Web. Whether you are raising your first toddler or your fourth teenager, you can find plenty of valuable information online. Many excellent Web sites blend professional advice, research, camaraderie, and fun into useful resources for parents and kids for your reading pleasure. This chapter helps you PILOT through the wealth of children's health Web sites and support groups, and guides you to the best sites where you and your kids can learn about their health.

Kids' Health for Parents

As a parent, you have questions about your child's health. What vaccinations does your child need? Is it just a cold, or is it something more serious? What can be done in the case of serious illness? And when you have healthy children—and you want them to stay that way—you want good advice on exercise, nutrition, and illness prevention.

A simple search on the keywords "parenting" or "kids' health" results in thousands of sites. These include experience-based personal pages, support, and information from other parents, magazine-like articles, and medical advice from pediatricians. As with all other health information on the Internet, use PILOT to evaluate the credibility of any site you surf.

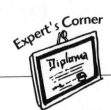

Treasures and Trash

"The Web is as much a medical breakthrough as any wonder drug. Parents (and kids!) can find virtually unlimited, free information, illustrations, and animations about every aspect of childhood health, development, diseases, and conditions. The challenge is that much of the health material on the Web is inaccurate, incomplete, out of date, overly commercial, or has an axe to grind. Yes, there are great health treasures on the Web, but families need to pick among the false jewels to find them. It is definitely worth the effort."

—Neil Izenberg, M.D., Director, Nemours Foundation Center for Children's Health Media, and Editor-in-Chief of KidsHealth.org

Researching Your Child's Illness Online

When your child is ill, whether it's a minor illness or a serious disease, you want answers, options, and support. The Internet can provide all three. Of course, you still need to consult with your pediatrician, but a little research on the Web can help you fully understand your child's ailment and arm you with knowledge when choosing treatment options. The following sites are good starting points.

KidSource

http://www.kidsource.com/kidsource/pages/health.diseases.html

This site provides you with a long list of excellent articles relating to pediatric illnesses, rated to help busy parents decide which ones to read first. These cover very specific conditions, such as back-to-school with food allergies, middle-ear fluid, and teen acne.

kidsDoctor

`http://www.kidsdoctor.com/`

Dr. Lewis A. Coffin III used to make house calls. Now he offers advice on kidsDoctor.com, "a 24-hour-a-day source for 'What every parent needs to know' when it comes to keeping our kids healthy." Topics are as varied as allergies, chicken pox, nosebleeds, bloody stools, smelly feet, and salty kisses.

Dr. Paula

`http://www.drpaula.com`

As colorful as your baby's nursery, this site gives you sound information from a friendly, informed pediatrician. Rashes, sleep, sore throat, Halloween safety, head lice, diarrhea, ear wax, and travel—whatever affects your child, you'll find information about it here, with dozens of articles written clearly and reassuringly (see Figure 11.1). Dr. Paula Elbirt practices at Mt. Sinai Medical Center in Manhattan.

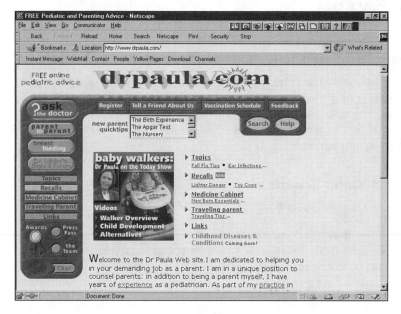

Figure 11.1

Pediatrician Dr. Paula gives advice to parents.

Virtual Children's Hospital: Pediatrics

`http://www.vh.org/VCH/Patients/Information.html`

The Children's Hospital of Iowa presents a varied and helpful assortment of patient information guides to children's illness, emergency information, and parenting tips. Each topic link leads to many different subtopics. For materials written *for* children, go to `http://www.vh.org/VCH/Patients/ForKids.html`.

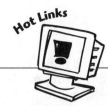

Facts for Families

http://www.aacap.org/publications/factsfam/index.htm

Health isn't solely physical. When children or adolescents display emotions or behavior that cause problems in their lives and the lives of others, this site provides insight. The American Academy of Child & Adolescent Psychiatry offers about 150 articles on a variety of emotional problems your child or teenager might be experiencing.

Parents Helping Parents

There's nothing quite like bringing your first baby home. It's a special time, indeed, but you are no doubt nervous and unsure of yourself. You can turn to other moms on the Internet who help answer your questions, commiserate, and share your joys.

It's a wonderful feeling to know that other parents are experiencing the same things you are. Whether you are a new mom or dad, your child is suffering from a serious illness, or you are struggling to control an independent teenager, you can be sure there are other parents out there who have "been there, done that." Check out these sites for great parent-to-parent support.

ParentsPlace.com Bulletin Boards

http://www.parentsplace.com/messageboards/

ParentsPlace is a terrific site that offers hundreds of bulletin boards dealing with every aspect of parenting, including more than 75 boards devoted to kids' health issues. Topics range from asthma to vaccines.

Children Today

http://childrentoday.com/

Children Today, a resource and community created to support parents of kids ages 6 through 9, is new from the iParenting folks who made Pregnancy Today so popular. Share online diaries and join Community Discussions where you connect with other parents who are going through the same issues as you. If your child is younger than 6, visit iParenting's Babies Today (http://babiestoday.com/) or Toddler's Today (http://toddlerstoday.com/).

Myria, the Magazine for Mothers

`http://www.myria.com/lists/`

Choose from more than 20 email discussion groups targeted to your child's age. You can also find a great number of resources on mothering topics.

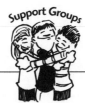

Parenting Newsgroups

In addition to the mailing lists and bulletin boards mentioned, try these newsgroups for parenting support:

➤ `misc.kids.health`   This active newsgroup covers all issues of kids' health.

➤ `alt.parent-teens`   This newsgroup provides support for people struggling with parent-teenager relationships.

➤ `misc.kids.pregnancy`   This newsgroup is a wonderful resource for pregnant and new moms.

Kids' Health for Kids

Let's not grab all the online fun and education for ourselves. Give the kids the keyboard, and let them explore these kid-friendly health information sites. Young Web surfers can ask questions and learn more about their growing bodies and personal health issues at the following sites.

KidsHealth.org for Kids

`http://kidshealth.org/kid/index.html`

How does your body work? What makes you sick? What keeps you safe? KidsHealth.org has fun and games to help kids learn about health.

Girl Power's BodyWise

`http://www.health.org/gpower/girlarea/bodywise/index.htm`

Targeted to girls aged 9 to 14, this friendly and colorful site offers tips on body image, nutrition, fitness, and sports, with special sections on eating disorders, diary excerpts from female Olympic athletes, and games and puzzles (see Figure 11.2).

Figure 11.2

Girl Power's BodyWise is "about learning to love and take care of your body."

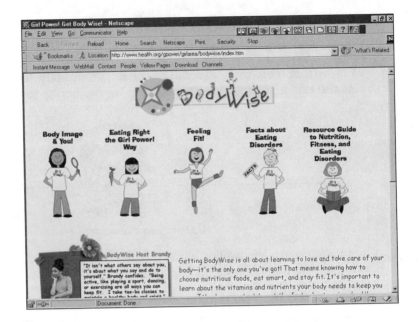

Band-Aides and Blackboards

http://funrsc.fairfield.edu/~jfleitas/contkids.html

With features such as "all about teasing," "hospital tour guides," and "pranks you can play in the hospital," this inspiring site helps kids deal with chronic illness and other medical problems.

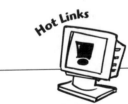

Hot Links

Healthy Fridge Kids' Quiz

http://www.healthyfridge.org/kids.html

Before you raid the refrigerator for some ice cream or soda, test your nutritional I.Q. with this "Healthy Fridge" quiz. As you answer each question correctly, your "fridge" fills up with nutritious foods!

Start Here: Healthy Kids' Web Sites

If you have children, these sites should be bookmarked in your browser!

KidsHealth.org

`http://kidshealth.org`

KidsHealth is a magnificent site that provides in-depth information on nutrition, fitness, emotions, safety, childhood infections, immunizations, and the latest treatments (see Figure 11.3). The site is split into three sections that effectively target parents, teens, and kids.

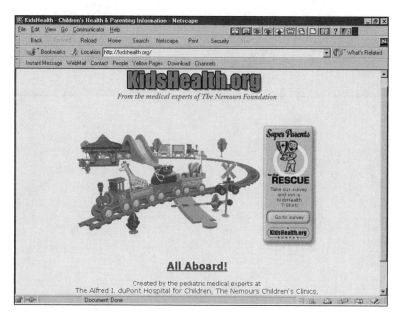

Figure 11.3

KidsHealth.org offers hundreds of articles for parents, teens, and kids. Click **All Aboard** *to read them.*

HealthyKids.com

`http://www.healthykids.com/`

HealthyKids.com is the online version of *Healthy Kids* magazine, a consumer publication of the American Academy of Pediatrics, so you're sure to find no-nonsense advice on everything from teething to temper tantrums. Choose from a bundle of message boards that put you in contact with parents who have children of the same age, single parents, parents considering adoption, or parents with special needs children.

ParentsPlace.com

`http://www.parentsplace.com/health/`

The Health section of ParentsPlace.com offers articles, Q&A, chats, and bulletin boards for illnesses, vaccines, development, safety, and even "adult" health concerns.

The Least You Need to Know

➤ Using the Internet, you can learn valuable information about your children's health, from your pregnancy through their adolescence.

➤ The Internet can guide you through a child's illness and provide support from other parents.

➤ Kids can have fun surfing the Web while learning about good health and fitness habits.

Part 4

Getting Well: Surgery, Drugs, and Alternatives

If you picked up this book, most likely you are in the midst of making choices that profoundly affect your health. Do you agree to a surgery that your doctor has recommended? What are the side effects of a particular drug, and how might it interact with your other medications? Are there non-invasive, alternative therapies that could help your condition?

The Internet has a wealth of information in these areas—and a lot of hogwash. The chapters in Part 4 help you cut through the hoaxes, gimmicks, advertisements, weirdness, and general confusion and open the path to solid, medically sound information.

And because addictions of all kinds are so devastating to users and everyone else who loves them or interacts with them, one chapter in Part 4 takes you to the best sites for getting unhooked from alcohol, drug, and tobacco addictions and eating disorders.

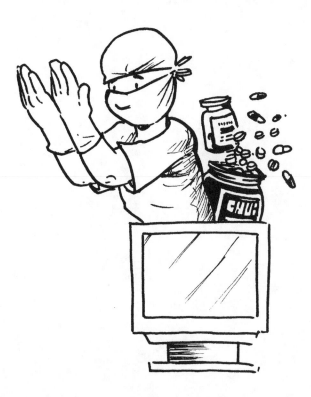

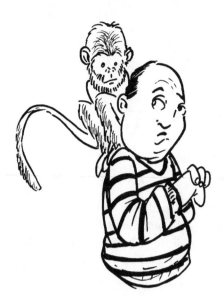

Chapter 12

Getting Unhooked: Fighting Addictions

In This Chapter

➤ Finding information about substance abuse online

➤ Identifying whether you have a drinking problem, and getting help

➤ Learning ways to quit smoking

➤ Educating yourself about eating disorders

➤ Getting support to help you quit an addiction

Drugs, alcohol, nicotine, eating disorders—addictions run rampant in our society, and there's nothing scarier than watching a loved one (or yourself!) self-destruct with addictive behavior. The Internet can't make an addiction magically disappear, but it can provide solid information, warning signs, motivation, and needed support. This chapter introduces you to some of the best sites for getting information and help.

Teens are at special risk for addictive behavior, because they experiment and consider themselves invulnerable to risk. So this chapter includes special sites targeted at teenagers and their parents.

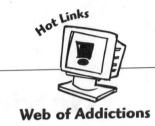

Web of Addictions

http://www.well.com/user/woa/

"We take addictions seriously. You won't find glib, hip treatment of this very serious topic here." This award-winning site has links, links, and more links to fact sheets, news, and support for drug, alcohol, and tobacco addictions, plus information on every drug you can think of. You could spend a week exploring all the links.

Drug Addiction

➤ 4.1 million people were hooked on illegal drugs in 1997 and 1998, according to the National Household Survey on Drug Abuse.

➤ About 25 percent of these drug abusers were only 12 to 17 years old.

➤ 3.7 million women have taken prescription drugs non-medically during the past year, according to the National Institute on Drug Abuse.

➤ More than 28,000 (70 percent) of the AIDS cases among women are drug related.

As you surf for information, realize that many sites have a strong point of view or agenda which might or might not fit with yours (take the issue of medical marijuana, for example). So if you're looking for "just the facts," make a point of separating the objective information from the subjective viewpoint.

If you or a loved one has a problem with drugs, the following sites can be your source of information, motivation, and support.

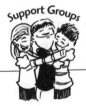

Recovery Works Support Resources

http://www.recovery-works.com/drugs.htm

This site has links to recovery sites, such as Narcotics Anonymous, Marijuana Anonymous, Cocaine Anonymous, and Chemically Dependent Anonymous.

Substance Abuse Center

http://onhealth.com/ch1/condctr/substance/item%2c51203.asp

This helpful and informative site from OnHealth is a terrific starting place because it gives the basics of reaching addiction, describes the highs and lows of major drugs of abuse, shows you how to recognize warning signs, discusses treatment options, and gives additional resources.

Drug-Free Resource Net

http://www.drugfreeamerica.org/

"The more you know about drugs, the more you can do to help the people you care about." This site from Partnership for a Drug-Free America offers a database of drug information, FAQs, and help for parents.

Principles of Drug Addiction Treatment: A Research-Based Guide

http://www.nida.nih.gov/PODAT/PODATindex.html

This detailed guide from the National Institutes of Health discusses how drug-addiction treatments benefit both the addict and society, explains the principles of effective treatment, and much more.

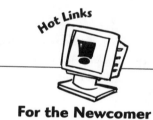

Hot Links

For the Newcomer

http://www.cdaweb.org/new.html

If you're new to 12-step programs, or considering getting into one, this welcoming guide from Chemically Dependent Anonymous answers your questions.

Freevibe

http://www.freevibe.com/

This hip, garishly colored site is aimed at youth. Click **heads up**, then **lowdown**, for strong anti-drug messages about the trendy drugs (for example: "Over time, steroid use can cause serious violent behavior, delusions, paranoid jealousy, and bad judgement. This is the kind of stuff that leads to suicide, murder, and general ruining-of-your-entire-life.")

Speakin' Out

`http://www.projectknow.com/A_teenspeak.html`

Kids and teens can read stories about the effects of drugs on families and friends. The stories are organized by theme, such as "Happy Endings," "Peer Pressure," and "Outta Control." "Not all the stories are happy ones. Some are sad and some are even scary. But all are real."

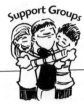

Web of Addictions Support Resources

`http://www.well.com/user/woa/aodsites.htm`

This collection of support resources from Web of Addictions includes self-help groups (and sites), mailing lists, and newsgroups for people with substance-abuse problems and professionals in the field.

Alcoholism

➤ As many as 6.6 million children live with at least one alcoholic parent.

➤ On a typical campus, the average amount a student spends on alcohol is $466 a year. Fifty percent of men and 39 percent of women college students in the United States are binge drinkers.

➤ Alcohol is associated with up to half of all traffic fatalities.

➤ About 1 million people were injured in alcohol-related crashes last year—an average of one injured every 30 seconds. About 30,000 people a year will suffer permanent work-related disabilities.

These statistics from *Generations Under the Influence* drive home what we already know: Alcoholism is a major addiction that hurts not only the alcoholic but his or her family, friends, and often total strangers.

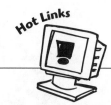

Generations Under the Influence

http://www.copleynewspapers.com/features/alcohol/

This superb, sobering 12-page report about our society's obsession with alcohol from the Copley newspaper chain combines emotionally charged photographs by Brian Plonka with moving stories by Denise Crosby.

Do You Have a Drinking Problem?

The following sites help you figure out whether it's time to get help for your drinking.

Self-Scoring Alcohol Check-up

http://www.habitsmart.com/chkup.html

"People vary tremendously in terms of how much they drink, why they drink and how drinking affects their lives." San Diego psychologist Robert W. Westermeyer, Ph.D., offers this brief, self-scoring test to learn whether your drinking is problematic enough to warrant changing it.

The Twenty Questions

http://www.recoveryresources.org/twenty.html

"Only you can decide if you have a 'drinking problem' and whether you want to do something about it." These 20 questions, presented by Sobriety and Recovery Resources, are used by many chemical dependency counselors in helping clients determine whether they have a problem with alcohol.

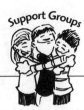

Support Sobriety and Recovery Resources

```
http://www.recoveryresources.org/
```

You'll never feel alone again if you follow these links to personal stories, articles, recovery sites, and online meetings, plus recovery links for other addictions.

Getting Help

After you've decided to get help, the Internet extends a helping hand seven days a week, 24 hours a day. Why not start with the best known organizations that can help you get and stay sober?

Al-Anon/Alateen

```
http://www.al-anon.alateen.org/
```

Al-Anon helps families and friends of alcoholics recover from the effects of living with the problem drinking of a relative or friend. Alateen is Al-Anon's recovery program for young people. Learn about both at this site.

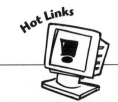

The Twelve Steps of Alcoholics Anonymous

```
http://www.
alcoholics-anonymous.org/
em24doc6.html
```

Here are A.A.'s famous Twelve Steps that guide members towards sobriety.

Alcoholics Anonymous

```
http://www.alcoholics-anonymous.org/
```

More than 2,000,000 A.A. members drank to excess in the past and then finally acknowledged that they could not handle alcohol, and now live a new way of life without it (see Figure 12.1). This site describes A.A.'s history, purpose, meetings, guidelines, and the Twelve Steps.

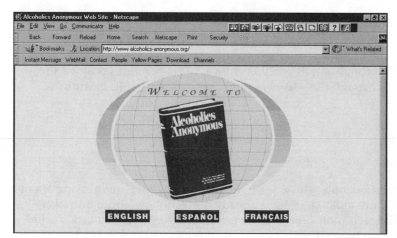

Figure 12.1

A.A. welcomes people who desire to stop drinking.

Kicking Butts: Smoking Cessation

"Tobacco is a custom loathsome to the eye, hateful to the nose, harmful to the brain, and dangerous to the lungs," declared King James I of England in 1604.

Each year, smoking kills more people than AIDS, alcohol, drug abuse, car crashes, murders, suicides, and fires combined! Tobacco use is the leading preventable cause of death in the United States, causing 400,000 deaths a year and resulting in $50 billion in direct medical costs and another $50 billion in indirect costs, according to the Centers for Disease Control (CDC).

Getting Motivated

Smokers might try to quit two, three, seven, or more times before they're successful. It's a powerful addiction, but half of all people who have ever smoked have quit—and you can be one of them, with online help.

Stop-Tabac.Ch

`http://www.stop-tabac.ch/en/documentation.html`

This site from the University of Geneva (Switzerland) has online brochures for people who have either firmly decided to stop smoking or are just considering it. Choose the one that fits your stage: precontemplation, contemplation, preparation, action, maintenance, or relapse.

Life After Cigarettes

http://www.quitnet.org/Library/Guides/ICQ/

"Quitting Smoking. The toughest job you'll ever love." This practical, positive site takes you by the hand through the reasons to quit, preparing to quit, quitting, and life after cigarettes.

Quitters

http://www.corral.net/quitters/

"This page is dedicated to people who want to quit smoking, who are thinking about quitting, are tying to quit smoking, or have already quit smoking" from a smoker who wanted to help himself quit. Learn all the reasons why you should kick, including a photo of a really nasty smoker's lung.

The QuitNet

http://www.quitnet.org/

"The QuitNet helps smokers kick their nicotine addiction. The 'Q' is not just a website. It is life support." This free service is provided by Join Together, a program of the Boston University School of Public Health. "The QuitNet is an online resource and support center for smokers struggling to quit and for those 'ex-smokers' working to stay quit." The QuitNet offers forums, chat, advice, guides, a personal mailbox, instant messaging, and buddy lists. There's no charge to use the service, but you have to register.

No-Smoke Cafe

http://www.clever.net/chrisco/nosmoke/cafe.html

"This here is the No-Smoke Cafe and this is YOUR home for as long as YOU want it to be. It's a place for anyone…young or old or in between can come if they have a desire to stop smoking or have already stopped smoking." If you wish you could hop over to a friendly, non-smoking coffee house and share a latte with friends as you engage in a spirited discussion about quitting smoking, this is your place, day or night (see Figure 12.2). Visit the **Self-Help Reading Library**, have a chat with a counselor, or peruse the message board. The special section called **Tips and Resources for the Newly Quit Smoker** offers "Quitmeters" (click to find out), Free Sticky Quit Note reminders, a certificate, and "The Wall of Ex-Smokers."

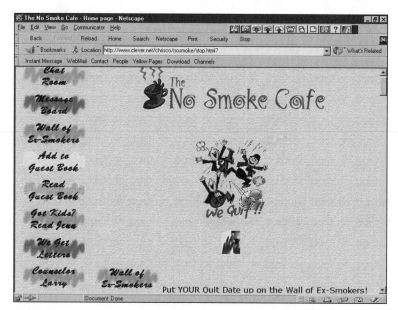

Figure 12.2

The No-Smoke Cafe is the ideal hangout for a surfer trying to quit smoking.

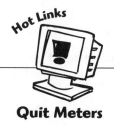

Hot Links

Quit Meters

Quit meters motivate you by letting you track the days and cigarettes you're not smoking. The following sites are sources for these tools:

➤ **QuitMeter** http://xnet2.com/quitmeter/ "One second at a time," the QuitMeter helps you quit smoking. You record your quit date, the usual number of cigarettes you smoke, and the price per pack. Then after you quit, the QuitMeter keeps track of all the cigarettes you didn't smoke and the money you didn't spend, and the length of time (to the second!) that you've been smoke-free. Really cool.

➤ **Quit Meters** http://quitsmoking.about.com/health/fitness/ quitsmoking/msubquitmeters.htm If you'd like to download a quit meter program instead of visiting it on the Web, here are links to about a dozen different free programs.

How to Quit

The following sites explain how to quit and help you do it.

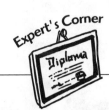

Commit to Quit

"Successful quitting is a matter of planning and commitment, not luck. Some options include using the nicotine patch or gum, joining a stop smoking class, going to Nicotine Anonymous meetings, or using self-help materials such as books and pamphlets."

—Ron Todd, Director, Tobacco Control, American Cancer Society

You Can Quit Smoking

http://www.ahcpr.gov/consumer/ch_quits.htm

Learn the three methods recommended by experts, according to the Agency for Health Care Policy and Research, and how you can put these methods into action.

Do You Smoke? Do You Want to Quit?

http://www.ahcpr.gov/consumer/smokecsm.htm

This practical site from the Agency for Health Care Policy and Research gives you strategies for quitting—including tips from other quitters—and explains why people who stop for good might quit more than once.

CDC's Tips: Tobacco Information and Prevention Source

http://www.cdc.gov/nccdphp/osh/tobacco.htm

"Warning: There is no safe tobacco product." This helpful site includes quick tobacco information and links, tobacco-related events in the news, Surgeon General's Reports related to tobacco, research, data, guides to help you quit, educational materials, and tips for kids and teens.

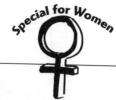

Special for Women

Women and Smoking

http://www.drkoop.com/wellness/tobacco/articles/women.asp

"Since the 1920s, the tobacco industry has targeted women with advertisements portraying smoking as liberating, glamorous, sexy, slenderizing, and feminine." Now almost 23 percent of adult American women smoke—about 22.6 million women. This article explores what science knows and doesn't know about women and tobacco.

Smoking and Your Health

http://www.healthlinkusa.com/385.htm

Treatments, cures, diagnosis, prevention, support groups, email lists, message boards, personal stories, risk factors, statistics, research, and more. The linked sites include Nicotine Anonymous on the Net, why you should quit, preparing yourself for quitting smoking, the effects of smoking on your lungs, and a "Stop Smoking Meter" that keeps track of how much you smoke and how much money you spend on tobacco products.

Smoking Cessation

http://quitsmoking.about.com/health/fitness/quitsmoking/

This extensive site from About.com has articles on every aspect of quitting smoking, plus many links to related topics from acupuncture to Zyban. Click **Smoking in Movies** to read the American Lung Association's movie ratings, a copy of Sylvester Stallone's agreement to smoke in films for $500,000, and a long list of celebrities who have died from smoking.

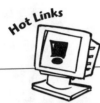

You KNEW These Folks

`http://quitsmoking.about.com/health/fitness/quitsmoking/msubmov.htm`

This list of dead celebrity puffers should make you grind out your cigarette on the spot. You probably knew Yul Brynner and John Wayne died of smoking-related diseases, but did you know about Judy Holiday, Mary Wells ("My Guy"), Burl Ives, Lee Remick, Walt Disney, Jack Benny, Nat "King" Cole, Lucille Ball, Desi Arnaz...the list goes on...and on.

Teen Smoking

These sobering statistics from the Centers for Disease Control should motivate you to help your favorite teenagers kick the tobacco habit:

➤ Most teen smokers believe they can quit, but after six years, 75 percent still smoke.

➤ Approximately 80 percent of adult smokers started smoking before the age of 18.

➤ Every day, nearly 3,000 young people under the age of 18 become regular smokers.

The following sites can help teens quit smoking or stick to a resolution never to start.

Tips 4 Teens

`http://www.cdc.gov/nccdphp/osh/tipsteen.htm`

The CDC presents motivating anti-smoking tip sheets and teen celebrity interviews. Be sure to click **Posters with a Message** to see some posters that will make your teen shudder.

American Cancer Society's Great American Smokeout

`http://www.cancer.org/smokeout`

"You Smoke You Choke!" This anti-smoking resource for students is colorful, entertaining, and clever (see Figure 12.3). The Smokeout is from the American Cancer Society.

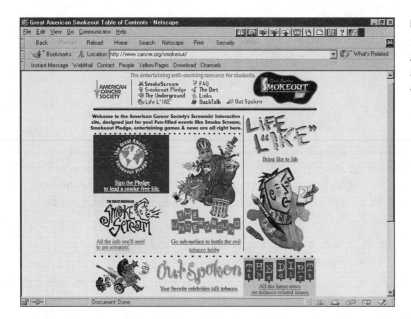

Figure 12.3

The Great American Smokeout entertains as much as it educates students.

The PATCH Project—Program Against Teen Chewing

http://www.patchproject.org/

Chewing and spitting tobacco seems cool to many male teens, but they might think twice after exploring this site, especially if they view the stomach-turning photos illustrating the disfigurement of oral cancer. The PATCH (Program Against Teen Chewing) Project, funded by the National Cancer Institute, aims to help adolescent males quit using spit tobacco (snuff or chewing tobacco).

NicNet

http://www.nicnet.org/

From the Arizona Program for Nicotine and Tobacco Research, Nicotine on the Net has links to all sorts of anti-tobacco sites by category, including cigars, pipes, chewing tobacco, kids, pregnancy, and environmental tobacco.

Tackling Tobacco

http://www.drkoop.com/wellness/tobacco/

This resource center for quitting tobacco has helpful articles, tools, message boards, and chats. Click **Tackling Tobacco Library** for articles on tobacco use and health; preparing to reduce/quit; ways to withdraw from nicotine; tackling cravings and relapse; and managing your feelings, stress, and weight.

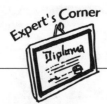

Chilling Statistics

"Today, nearly 3,000 young people across our country will begin smoking regularly. Of these 3,000 young people, 1,000 will lose that gamble to the diseases caused by smoking. The net effect of this is that among children living in America today, 5 million will die an early, preventable death because of a decision made as a child."

—Donna E. Shalala, Ph.D., Secretary, U.S. Department of Health and Human Services (from `http://www.cdc.gov/nccdphp/osh/oshaag.htm`)

TobaccoFree.Org

`http://www.tobaccofree.org/`

The Foundation for a Smokefree America was founded by R.J. Reynolds's wayward grandson, Patrick Reynolds, who talks to teens and kids about staying tobacco-free and resisting the tobacco advertising and peer pressure. (Patrick Reynolds's father and grandfather died of tobacco-related diseases after making their fortunes by hooking smokers.) This site has the text of his powerful speeches (including artwork of great cigarette-ad parodies) and quitting tips for adults, as well as teens.

Question It

`http://www.questionit.com/`

"Tobacco is the only legal product that, when used as recommended, results in death." This hip site encourages teens to "get pissed, get moving, and get wise about tobacco addiction." Be sure to read **Tricks of the Trade** to learn how the cigarette companies get smokers addicted quickly.

Eating Disorders

Is your weight-loss goal self-destructive?

➤ The average North American woman wears size 14.

➤ A typical model weighs less than 75 percent of an average woman's weight. This used to be 92 percent.

➤ More than 11 million North American females suffer from eating disorders.

➤ Fifty percent of adolescents are trying to lose weight.

➤ Fifty percent of fourth graders have dieted.

"But I'm so fat!" Our society's fixation on weight loss can lead to an eating disorder, such as anorexia nervosa (self-starvation while still seeing oneself as fat), bulimia (bingeing and vomiting), or obsessive overeating. These sites can help you recognize and understand eating disorders, and help someone who has one.

Eating Disorders

http://www.massmed.org/community/hinfo/overeat/index.html

This guide from the Massachusetts Medical Society has separate articles for parents and teens on anorexia, bulimia, and compulsive eating.

BodyWise

http://www.health.org/gpower/girlarea/bodywise/

BodyWise is a site for girls. Click **Facts about Eating Disorders** for articles that explain these disorders clearly and compassionately, in terms even young teens will understand. Colorful cartoons add to the attractiveness of this site (see Figure 12.4).

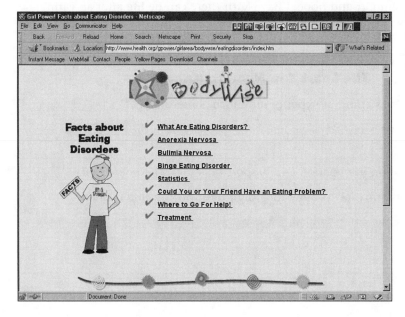

Figure 12.4

Girls can learn about eating disorders at the BodyWise Web site.

General Information on Eating Disorders

http://www.aabainc.org/general/index.html

Read explanations of the different types of eating disorders, warning signs, and medical consequences from the American Anorexia Bulimia Association, Inc.

Eating Disorders Awareness and Prevention, Inc.

http://members.aol.com/edapinc/

This national not-for-profit organization is dedicated to increasing the awareness and prevention of eating disorders, with programs and an instructive Web site. EDAP aims to educate people about eating disorders and eliminate the 3 Ds: body dissatisfaction, dieting behavior, and drive for thinness. There are articles for parents, teens, kids, and friends.

The Something Fishy Web Site on Eating Disorders

http://www.something-fishy.org/

Amy, a member of the Something Fishy band, had anorexia. As she and her husband learned more about the disorder and how to cope with it, they started accumulating information for this Web site. It has grown into a large, informative site about all types of eating disorders, with a warm and personal touch. "If we can continue to come together with support and hope, I have faith there can be life after an eating disorder," writes Amy.

The Least You Need to Know

➤ You can get facts about all types of substance abuse online.

➤ The Internet has a myriad of resources for recovery from drug or alcohol abuse.

➤ Smoking cessation information and support online can help you quit.

➤ If you need information about eating disorders, you can find it online.

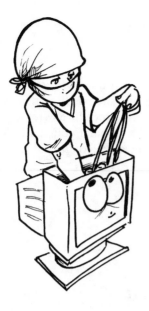

Chapter 13

Surgery

In This Chapter

➤ Learning about a surgical procedure online

➤ Getting the facts about preparing for surgery

➤ Exploring cosmetic surgery

➤ Learning about transplants

Seventy million people in the United States face surgery each year. If you're one of them, the more you can learn about your surgery ahead of time, the more easily your doctor can educate you about the benefits and risks and the procedure itself. Nothing dispels fear like knowledge, and this chapter shows you where you can learn about your surgery online.

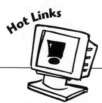

Hot Links

Medicine Online: Bid for Surgery

http://www.medicineonline.com/bid4surgery

Good grief, it's a surgery auction. Surgeons bid on the opportunity to perform your next elective surgical procedure. Only elective cosmetic, foot and ankle, or vision-correcting surgery qualifies. Is this really weird, or is it the future of free-market medicine? Would you want your facelift done by the lowest bidder?

What Can You Learn Online?

After your doctor, the World Wide Web is your next best resource for surgery information. As long as you get your content from a reputable site, such as the ones recommended here, you can get up-to-date knowledge about the procedure, why it is done, how it is done (in as much graphic detail as you want!), and what you can expect afterwards. You can view medical illustrations, photos, even video clips of the procedure.

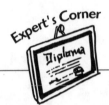

Information Versus Medicine

"Just as a sharp scalpel does not alone make a good surgeon, access to information does not itself translate into the best medicine. While the Internet can provide a great deal of knowledge—you might find details about 50 ways to perform breast biopsy—how do you know what's best for you and your needs? No Internet site can replace the physician's experience and understanding of your specific history, nor can information from the Net supplant the relationship between patient and doctor in determining what is the best treatment path for you. Only the surgeon, working with an individual patient, can decide whether and how to operate—not the scalpel."

—Dr. Eric Whitacre, M.D., F.A.C.S., Breast Surgeon, The Breast Center at Mercy Medical Center, Baltimore, Maryland

Start Here: Surgical Procedure Sites

The following sites give you anywhere from a quick overview to an in-depth explanation of a variety of surgical procedures.

HealthAnswers

`http://healthanswers.com`

Click **Find a surgical procedure** under Find It Quickly, and then find the procedure that interests you in the alphabetical "surgical procedure finder." HealthAnswers gives you a guide to that surgery, including definition, description, indications, expectations after surgery, convalescence, risk, and cost. Photos enhance your understanding. This is a handy place to start.

PreOp.com

http://www.preop.com

PreOp.com helps you understand the surgical procedure most commonly used to treat a specific medical condition. Read the **Welcome** introduction, and then click **General Public** for a procedure list, including Achilles tendon repair, meniscus (knee) repair, spleen removal, and general open surgery. Each procedure presents information in text, illustrations, and video and audio clips. (At press time, a number of procedures were still under production.)

MedicineNet.com

http://www.medicinenet.com/

Click **Procedures & Tests** at the top, and then find the surgery you want from the alphabetical list. You find a "start here" main article and related information.

Herbs and Surgery

"If you take herbs, be especially careful if you're headed into surgery. It is standard medical practice to ask pre-operative patients about prescription drugs or even over-the-counter drugs like aspirin. But few anesthesiologists think to ask patients which herbs they take. Ginkgo biloba, garlic, glucosamine, and ginger can easily interfere with bleeding, sedation, or blood pressure. Several patients have already gotten into trouble. You don't have to give up your herbs forever, just stop taking them several weeks before surgery—and make sure you tell your doctor."

—Dean Edell, M.D., author of *Eat, Drink & Be Merry* (www.healthcentral.com)

Some Common Surgeries

Detailing the surgeries you can learn about online would take a whole book in itself. The following sites teach you about some common surgeries. If the one you're seeking isn't listed, find it at the sites listed previously in "Start Here: Surgical Procedure Sites," or enter it as a search word at `http://www.healthfinder.gov/`.

Coronary Artery Bypass Graft (CABG) Surgery

`http://www.medicinenet.com/`

Click **Procedures & Tests** at the top, find **heart bypass** in the alphabetical list, and then select **Coronary Artery Bypass Graft** under **main article**. Coronary artery bypass graft (CABG) surgery (commonly known as heart bypass) is one of the most commonly performed major operations in the United States—about 350,000 times a year. Learn about this operation (and about coronary artery disease) in this detailed guide from MedicineNet.com.

Questions and Answers about Hip Replacement

`http://www.nih.gov/niams/healthinfo/hiprepqa.htm`

Hip replacement surgery improves mobility and relieves pain in people whose hip joints are wearing down, often due to osteoarthritis. This site from the National Institute of Arthritis and Musculoskeletal and Skin Diseases gives an overview of this operation.

Hysterectomy: Removal of the Uterus

`http://www.preop.com`

Click **General Public**, **Hysterectomy—Removal of Uterus**. If you're having (or considering having) a hysterectomy, PreOp.com tells you everything about it. Click the items at the left to learn what a hysterectomy is (with anatomical illustrations), alternatives, anesthesia, before surgery, the procedure, and recovery. This site includes video and audio clips.

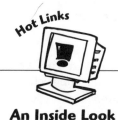

An Inside Look

Have you wished you could peek at what lies under the skin of the human body? Here are a few sites that make that possible:

➤ `http://www.nlm.nih.gov/research/visible/visible_gallery.html`
Visible Human Project Gallery from the National Library of Medicine shows you movies of cryosections—anatomically detailed slices of an area of the human body.

➤ `http://www.healthcentral.com/drdean/deanfulltexttopics.cfm?id=20773`
Plastination Photos: Anatomy Art from Dr. Dean Edell's HealthCentral is an introduction to the art of plastination, a process that allows for the preservation of entire human bodies, including individual tissues, organs, and organ systems in a lifelike way. Click **more of these fascinating photos** to view more in this series.

➤ `http://www.plastination.com/english/plastination.htm` The Plastination site from the Institut für Plastination in Heidelberg teaches you about this fascinating process. Click all the topics that interest you.

Preparing for Surgery

As you decide to have surgery and prepare for it, a million questions occur to you that you didn't think (or didn't have time) to ask your doctor. The following sites help you prepare for surgery and answer your questions. (In fact, do your doctor the favor of making sure he or she knows about these sites to recommend them to other patients!)

Sizing Up Surgery

http://www.fda.gov/fdac/features/1998/698_surg.html

"Whether you are undergoing surgery for the first time or the tenth, understanding why you need it, the risks involved, available alternative treatments, and the after-effects will help you make the right decisions and deal effectively with the outcome." This article from *FDA Consumer* discusses the value of a second opinion, routine laboratory tests, anesthesia, risks of infection, and questions to ask your doctor before you have surgery.

When You Need an Operation

http://www.facs.org/

Click **Public Information, When You Need an Operation** for guidelines from the American College of Surgeons about choosing a surgeon, seeking a consultation, giving informed consent, and learning the costs.

Anesthesia Net

http://anesthesia.net/

If you're preparing for surgery, Anesthesia Net helps you understand the experience of anesthesia. Click **A Typical Experience** to read a patient's guide to anesthesia with a step-by-step explanation of how you will be prepared for anesthesia, the different types, and the post-anesthesia experience.

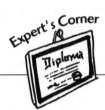

Expert's Corner

Be Informed: Questions to Ask Your Doctor Before You Have Surgery

The Agency for Health Care Policy and Research (AHCPR) recommends asking your surgeon the following questions. (For more information about each question, read the guide at http://www.ahcpr.gov/consumer/surgery.htm.)

1. What operation are you recommending?
2. Why do I need the operation?
3. Are there alternatives to surgery?
4. What are the benefits of having the operation?
5. What are the risks of having the operation?
6. What if I don't have this operation?
7. Where can I get a second opinion?
8. What has been your experience in doing the operation?
9. Where will the operation be done?
10. What kind of anesthesia will I need?
11. How long will it take me to recover?
12. How much will the operation cost?

Viewing Surgery Online

Okay, sometimes it's not enough just to *read* about a surgical procedure—you want to see it! Carnie Wilson opened the public's eyes by having her gastric bypass surgery transmitted online. If you don't want to get that graphic, you can view medical artwork that shows you what the affected body parts look like, and what the surgeon does to them.

Whether your interest is educational or voyeuristic, you can find sites to satisfy your hungry eye.

Adam.com's Health Illustrated

`http://www.adam.com/health_illustrated/health_illustrated.htm`

"A picture is worth a thousand words." Adam.com's Health Illustrated series features award-winning, full-color medical artwork of more than 45 surgeries "far beyond what words alone could describe." These vivid illustrations show the anatomy of your problem and what your surgeon might do to correct it (see Figure 13.1). Choose the procedure, and then click the circled numbers above the first illustration to see more. A fascinating site!

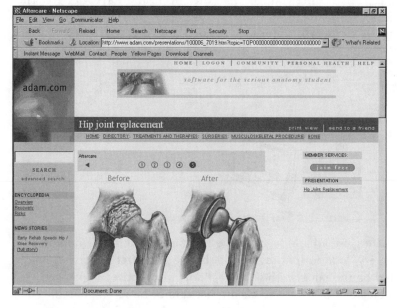

Figure 13.1

Adam.com Health Illustrated shows "before and after" illustrations of hip replacement surgery.

A Doctor in Your House

`http://www.adoctorinyourhouse.com/`

Did you miss Carnie Wilson's gastric bypass surgery? Watch the archived video, or, if that makes you shudder, watch videos of other celebrities discussing their surgeries and ailments. This site describes itself as "celebrity driven healthcare information, designed to inform, empower and entertain."

Cyber Surgery Suite

`http://thehealthnetwork.com/liveevents/archive.asp`

View Webcasts of surgeries and other medical procedures at TheHealthNetwork.com's Cyber Surgery Suite while doctors describe what is happening. "This is the reality of medical care behind the wide, swinging doors where family members may not go."

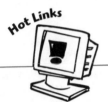

Hot Links

American Society for Dermatologic Surgery

`http://www.asds-net.org/`

Chemical peels, tattoo removal, skin cancer, scar removal—if a dermatologic (skin) surgeon performs the procedure, you can learn about it here.

Cosmetic Surgery

Every year, more than two million people change their looks through cosmetic surgery. Whether it's nose shape, breast size, or eyelid sag, people are altering those parts of their faces and bodies that make them self-conscious.

"Rejuvenation" surgery is especially popular right now. From baby boomers to sprightly seniors, people are feeling younger than their years and staying active. The demand for cosmetic surgery—especially eyelid surgery, facelifts, liposuction, and laser skin resurfacing—is soaring, according to the American Society of Plastic Surgeons. If you're considering cosmetic surgery, check out the following sites first.

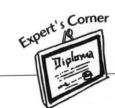

Expert's Corner

Cosmetic Surgery Cautions

"Many doctor's sites are glorified ads, high on the glitz factor and short on information. In plastic surgery, look for photographs of before and after surgery patients. Views should be the same, with similar lighting, perspective, angles, hair, and makeup. Be careful of hype and claims that cannot be substantiated. Remember the Internet does not replace the office consultation. Only a doctor who has examined the problem can properly advise you about risks, benefits, and alternate methods of care."

—Michael Bermant, M.D., plastic surgeon (`http://www.plasticsurgery4u.com`)

Plastic Surgery Information Services

`http://www.plasticsurgery.org/`

This site, sponsored by the American Society of Plastic Surgeons (ASPS) and the Plastic Surgery Educational Foundation (PSEF), offers information on a variety of cosmetic and reconstructive surgery procedures and includes a plastic-surgeon referral service. Read a quick overview under **Procedures at a Glance**, or go into detail by reading full articles, complete with illustrations.

E-sthetics

`http://www.phudson.com/`

This site from plastic surgeon Patrick Hudson, M.D., presents information about many cosmetic surgeries, including facelift, liposuction, breast enlargement, abdominoplasty (tummy tuck), facial sculpturing, body sculpturing, and scar revision, with before and after photos.

Bermant Plastic and Cosmetic Surgery

`http://www.plasticsurgery4u.com/`

Plastic surgeon Michael Bermant, M.D., offers more than 300 pages of information on reconstructive, hand, cosmetic, congenital, breast, head and neck, and skin cancer surgeries, with plenty of articles, before and after photos (including injured children), and surgical details. Check out Dr. Bermant's artwork, too.

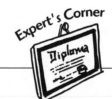

Expert's Corner

Wear Your Seatbelt

"I have spent hours picking pieces of glass from the multiple lacerations people get when their faces impact against the windshield."

—Michael Bermant, M.D., plastic surgeon (`http://www.plasticsurgery4u.com`)

Surgery.Com

`http://www.surgery.com/`

"Improve your body image, and feel better." Learn about breast implants, laser surgery, hair transplant, liposculpture, facelifts, and breast reconstruction; see before and after photos; and locate plastic surgeons in your area.

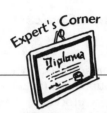

Plastic Surgery Cautions

"Be careful about Web sites that are soliciting plastic surgery patients. Review the site critically. Make sure there is a doctor with a direct link to answer questions. The doctor should answer your questions personally and in a reasonable period of time and have his or her credentials clearly visible and in detail. The doctor should be willing to answer any questions including those about lawsuits. Only when these criteria are met would I consider the information and resources to be trustworthy."

—James J. Romano, M.D., cosmetic surgeon (`http://www.jromano.com`)

Transplants

The first (failed) organ-transplantation experiments were done on animals and humans in the 18th century. By the mid-20th century, successful organ transplants had been performed. Now transplants of kidneys, livers, hearts, pancreases, lungs, and heart-lungs are an accepted part of medical treatment, according to the United Network for Organ Sharing (`http://www.unos.org`).

Are you a candidate? Are you interested in getting on the list? Donating an organ? The Internet is your pipeline to information about transplants and donations.

TransWeb: All About Transplant and Donation

`http://TransWeb.org`

Planning an organ transplant or donation? Have you had one? Are you waiting for one? Just curious? This award-winning site is an exceptional resource with 10,000 items, including FAQs, details about organ donations, news, personal accounts, lifestyle information, and links to transplant centers. Click **The Transplant Journey** for a multimedia guide to the transplant process (see Figure 13.2).

Transplant Living

`http://www.unos.org/patients/`

"Every 16 minutes a new name is added to the national organ transplant waiting list." This site from the United Network for Organ Sharing (UNOS) has an online database for checking transplant statistics at different centers and for different organs. Read **Transplant 101** about getting on the list, financing, and life after transplant.

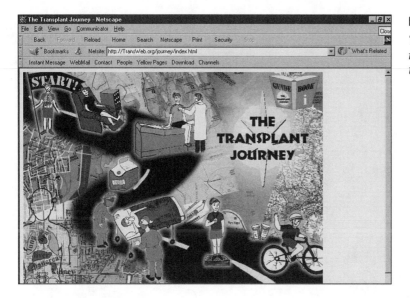

Figure 13.2

TransWeb takes you on a multimedia tour of the transplant process.

The Least You Need to Know

➤ The Web has resources for learning about how and why various surgeries are performed.

➤ You can view videos, drawings, and photos of surgeries online.

➤ Web sites help prepare you for surgery by explaining what to expect.

➤ Making a decision about cosmetic surgery is easier when you read about the procedures and see photos on the Web.

➤ You can learn about transplants and track activity at different centers online.

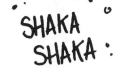

SHAKA
SHAKA

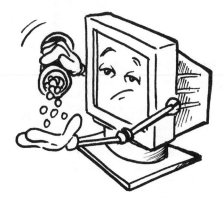

Chapter 14

Medications and Supplements

In This Chapter

➤ Finding information about prescription drugs

➤ Exploring herbal medicine

➤ Buying drugs online

➤ Understanding the risks of self-medication and drug interactions

The World Wide Web is a powerful source of medication information. You can look up any drug—prescription, over-the-counter, or herbal—and find out everything about it, including uses, clinical studies, side effects, interactions with other drugs, and contraindications (circumstances when this drug is not advised). Several sites even put this information into plain English! And if you want, you can order the medications you need right from the computer without changing out of your pajamas and fuzzy slippers.

This chapter shows you how to get good medication info by steering you toward reputable sites and bringing some caveats to your attention.

Rx Online

The Internet is revolutionizing what consumers know about and how they purchase medications. This is good and bad. It's good because an educated consumer is more likely to get better care. It's bad because the regulations and safeguards that minimize risk when you get your prescriptions filled at your local pharmacy are easily circumvented in cyberspace.

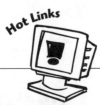

Hot Links

Questions All Patients Should Ask Their Pharmacist About Their Medications

http://www.pueblo.gsa.gov/cic_text/health/askpharmacist/
ask-pharmacist.htm

Print out these 10 questions to ask your pharmacist from the American Pharmaceutical Association and take them with you when you fill your next prescription.

What Can You Learn?

One of the most satisfying medical uses of the World Wide Web is the ease of learning the facts about medications you're taking, considering taking, or just curious about. Whether you're comfortable reading medical lingo or need it translated into lay person's language, you can find accurate, up-to-date information online. Learn what drugs are used to treat your condition and how they should be taken. Read the side effects, and check out alternatives. The more familiar you are with the facts, the more intelligently you can talk with your doctor or pharmacist. And the more information you have, the more solid your foundation is for making choices about medications.

After you've done some reading, you might need professional advice to make sense of it. A number of sites have pharmacists who answer questions online. This can be very helpful in educating yourself about the benefits and risks of certain drugs and appropriate treatments for particular medical treatments in general, sometimes including complementary treatments.

But realize that as smart and well-educated as online pharmacists and physicians might be, they don't know you, don't know what other medications you're taking, and have never examined you, asked you questions, or read your medical history. So, take the advice as general information, but consult your own health professional to ensure it applies to you.

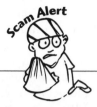

Scam Alert

Internet Availability of Prescription Pharmaceuticals to the Public

http://www.acponline.org/journals/annals/05oct99/bloom.htm

This study from Annals of Internal Medicine investigated the price and ease of obtaining certain prescription drugs on the Internet. You might be surprised to learn that ordering online costs an average of 10 percent more than ordering at your local pharmacy, and that's before adding on a hefty shipping charge. Many online pharmacies issued prescriptions after a "consultation" where the buyer filled out a questionnaire—and sometimes the "correct" choices were preselected! Of the 46 sites studied, nine (all based outside of the United States) required neither a prescription nor a consultation.

Buying Prescription Drugs Online

After you have a prescription for a medication, you can get it filled online. The e-pharmacy walks you through the process for getting your prescription transferred, and its pharmacist checks it. Be aware that some insurance companies do not pay for online drug purchases, so look into this before you order.

How do you know whether the online pharmacy you've chosen is reputable? Look for the VIPPS (Verified Internet Pharmacy Practice Sites) seal, being introduced by the National Association of Boards of Pharmacy to identify licensed sites in good standing. You can also be sure the seal is authentic by checking with the National Association of Boards of Pharmacy at http://www.nabp.net. Click **VIPPS**, and then **VIPPS list**.

No Prescription, No Drug

Understand that reputable online pharmacies will fill prescriptions and provide over-the-counter drugs, but they won't provide prescription drugs when you *don't* have a prescription. This makes sense—if a medication is powerful enough to be classified prescription-only, then you should get it only after a health professional has examined you, checked your medical history, and determined that this treatment is warranted.

However, it's very easy to find disreputable or foreign sites that are willing to sell you prescription drugs without a prescription. Especially popular drugs at these sites are

Viagra for sexual potency, Propecia for hair growth, Prozac for depression, and Xenical for weight loss. You have an online "examination" or "consultation" by answering a few questions, and zip, you've got a prescription. Obviously, you (or a teenager in your household) could say anything—exaggerate a condition, make up a condition—as long as the credit card number is authentic. This is dangerous—no one can evaluate whether you should get a powerful drug by collecting a few survey answers. Please help stamp out these dangerous practices by not supporting them.

Self-Medication: Risky Business

Even when the drug or herb you want to buy is available without a prescription, self-medication has the potential to be dangerous. You don't know the most current information about the drug you're considering, how it works for your medical condition, how it might interact with other drugs you're taking, and how it might affect your other medical conditions. So, don't start, stop, or cut back on a medication without consulting your physician or pharmacist. What you don't know *can* hurt you.

Investigating Online Pharmacies

If you do have a prescription for a medication, the convenience and privacy of ordering online might appeal to you, especially if the last thing you want to do is stand in line with your neighbors picking up a prescription for a sensitive condition. Here are some questions to explore to make your e-pharmacy experience a safe and happy one:

- ➤ What free information does the site provide that is not geared towards sales? What unbiased information can you find out about your medication before you buy it?

- ➤ Does the site require a prescription from a physician or authorized health-care provider? (The reputable ones do.)

- ➤ What are the credentials of the pharmacists on staff? Can you ask questions of a registered pharmacist at any hour?

- ➤ What are the shipping and handling costs? Are you really saving money? If not, is the convenience worth the extra cost?

- ➤ Is the e-pharmacy licensed in your state? Each state has its own guidelines and regulations. The most reputable sites only sell to you if they are licensed in your state.

- ➤ How is the site protecting your privacy? Who gets access to your records? What safeguards prevent snoops?

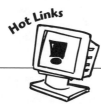

Confessions of an Online Drug User

`http://www.upside.com/texis/mvm/story?id=37839bc30`

Can you fill your prescriptions through the online drugstores, get your insurance to pay, and save money? Yes, no, and yes, found writer Robert McGarvey in this lively article.

Reputable e-Pharmacies

Here are some reputable e-pharmacies. Compare prices, policies, and access to a pharmacist for your questions:

➤ **CVS.com (formerly soma.com)** `http://www.CVS.com` (see Figure 14.1)

➤ **Drug Emporium** `http://www.drugemporium.com`

➤ **Drugstore.com** `http://www.drugstore.com`

➤ **Familymeds.com** `http://www.familymeds.com`

➤ **PlanetRx** `http://www.planetrx.com`

➤ **Rx.com** `http://www.Rx.com`

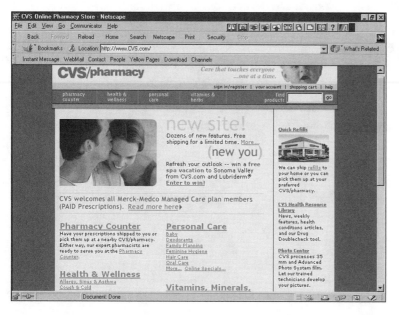

Figure 14.1

CVS.com is an online pharmacy for prescription and over-the-counter drugs, and supplements.

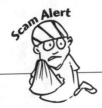

False Tenets of Paraherbalism

http://www.quackwatch.com/01QuackeryRelatedTopics/paraherbalism.html

Read these 10 tips for spotting pseudoscientific claims for herbs by Varro E. Tyler, Ph.D., former Lilly distinguished professor of pharmacognosy (the science of medicines from natural sources) at Purdue University.

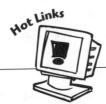

Medical Marijuana

Should medical marijuana be legal? Get the facts about this hot topic at the following sites:

➤ **Medical Marijuana Center**, http://www.healthcentral.com/Centers/OneCenter.cfm?Center=Marijuana   Read several articles and news reports from Dr. Dean Edell on the topic of medical marijuana.

➤ **Medicinal Marijuana Facts**, http://www.mpp.org/mmjfacts.html   This fact sheet gives statistics about the support of medical marijuana from the public, physicians, and medical organizations, along with arrest stats.

➤ **Marijuana and Medicine: Assessing the Science Base**, http://www.mpp.org/science.html   What medical conditions are helped by marijuana? Why not just use Marinol in pill form? If patients were allowed to use medicinal marijuana, wouldn't overall use increase? This site answers these questions and many more, although in very formal language.

Herbal Medicine

Herbs—plants that are used for medicinal purposes—are big news. We hear their impressive benefits proclaimed by national newspapers, radio talk shows, health-food stores, and our friends. We're taking herbal supplements for a bevy of conditions, including PMS, weight loss, depression, and memory loss. There's something comforting and natural about brewing an aromatic herb tea to treat an ailment rather than popping a pill. But realize that herbs *are* medicine, and should not be used willy-nilly. Educate yourself using the Internet, but be aware—you probably are getting tired of hearing this—that there's a lot of misinformation out there.

Herbal Mix Alert

Fifty percent of adult Americans are using herbal medicines, and 70 percent of those don't tell their doctor. Mixing herbs with other medications and conditions can be a recipe for disaster because of therapeutic interactions. For example, garlic can lower blood sugar, which is a caution in diabetes. Ginkgo can increase the effect of blood-thinning medications in an erratic manner. Some herbs can worsen certain medical conditions, such as saw palmetto, which can aggravate prostate cancer. Some herbs should be avoided if you are pregnant or nursing. So, talk to your doctor or pharmacist about any herbs you're considering taking.

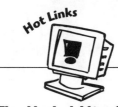

Hot Links

The Herbal Minefield

http://www.quackwatch.com/01QuackeryRelatedTopics/herbs.html

This article from Quackwatch.com tells you why you have to be careful about buying herbs to treat medical conditions: The active ingredients (with the medical properties you want) are not standardized, contents and potency are not accurately disclosed, side effects and safety might not be known or disclosed, and they might be sold by people who don't know what they're talking about.

Herbs Online

You'll find lots of herb sites on the Web—some are out to sell you and some are out to snow you, but the following sites provide substantial information. It's a good idea to check herbal information in more than one site, because few sites have everything right and up to date.

AllHerb.com

`http://www.allherb.com`

Although this site is an herbal store, the information here is in-depth and invaluable. You'll find a complete reference of herbs, vitamins, minerals, and supplements (see Figure 14.2). Click **The Basics** for plain-English primers on herbs, alternative medicine, vitamins, and nutrition.

Figure 14.2

AllHerb.com offers a user-friendly site full of herbal, alternative, and nutritional information.

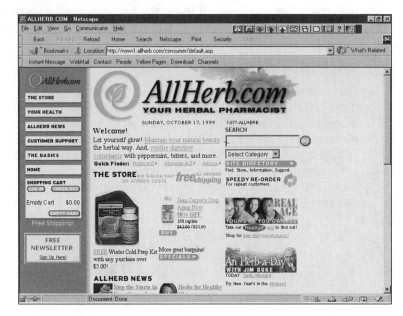

The Herb Research Foundation

`http://www.herbs.org`

Scientific, political, and business news on herbal medicine. The "Online Greenpapers" highlight specific herbs and their medicinal uses.

HerbMed

`http://www.amfoundation.org/herbmed.html`

This research-based, comprehensive site enables you to look up any herb and learn all about it, including medical uses, clinical data, toxic and adverse effects, interactions, traditional and folk use, suppliers, pictures, and plenty of scientific information. If the scientific language is daunting, take a printout to your health provider. This site does not sell products.

Healthwell.com

http://www.healthwell.com

Look up "Pharmacy" in the Health and Healing Index to read articles on herbs, supplements, herb-drug interactions, vitamins, minerals, and Western medicine. This site provides a good variety of herb articles and interesting tidbits.

Medicine Cabinet

http://medicinecabinet.net/

Click **Encyclopedia**, then **Herbs**, for solid, science-backed information on the medicinal qualities of about 200 herbs, including the scientific references. Or click **Diseases & Conditions**, **Nutritional Supplements**, **Homeopathy**, or **Diets & Therapies** for more natural-health information.

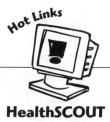

HealthSCOUT

http://www.healthscout.com

Scroll down to **Directory** and click **Alternative Medicine**, and then **Herbal Medicine**. You'll find about 30 interesting news articles about herbal medicine, with titles as intriguing as "Garlic Breath (why mints fail)" and "Nipping Roaches in the Bud (catnip repels cockroaches)."

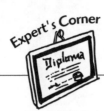

Advice from the Pharmacist

➤ **Don't buy prescription drugs online when you don't have a prescription.** These medications are prescription for a reason—they are not safe for unsupervised use! Severe side effects can ruin your life. Ask the pro football player who went into kidney failure from too much prescription-strength ibuprofen.

➤ **Tell the online pharmacist everything else you're taking.** The pharmacist needs to check for drug interactions. Along with your prescription, provide a list of all medications, OTC drugs, nutritional supplements, and herbal medications you are taking. (Take this list with you when you go to see your doctor, too!) If you use a site with no pharmacist, you are playing Russian roulette.

➤ **Ask, "Is there anything else I can do that might help?"** Do this when you're consulting a pharmacist, either online or live, about a treatment for a medical condition. Often pharmacists can recommend nontraditional treatments, such as a stress reduction class for stomach ailments.

➤ **Stick to reliable herb sites.** Otherwise, it's a crap shoot. Most sites have some good information mixed in with unreliable and often downright dangerous information. How many sites tell you not to take hawthorn products with some heart medications, for example? Do they warn about avoiding certain herbs in pregnancy/lactation? Do they list side effects? Too often, they list so many uses that you don't know the herb's common use.

➤ **Be a shrewd consumer of herbs, online and offline.** Unless you have a knowledgeable healthcare practitioner on your side, you must educate yourself about how your herbal medicines (yes, they are medicine!) will interact with your other medications and/or medical conditions. Also be wary of the product quality. One study of Asian/Korean ginseng products in North America found that 50 percent had no ginseng in them at all! Stick to the recognized brand names. They usually cost a little more, but you are worth it!

—Paul Roberts, R.Ph., clinical pharmacist at Kaiser Permanente in Santa Rosa, CA

©1999 Paul Roberts, R.Ph.

Vitamins and Minerals

What vitamins and minerals do we need? How much? Which foods contain them? Do we have to take supplements? The Web has unlimited vitamin information. It also has unlimited pseudo-information, too—so please remember our PILOT Method! Here are some good sites that can answer all your questions.

Vitamin and Nutritional Supplements

http://www.mayohealth.org/mayo/9707/htm/me_jun97.htm

The nutritional supplement industry is a $6-billion-a-year business. This article from the Mayo Clinic's Health Oasis sorts fact from fiction and helps you cut through the hype to understand just what you need and why.

Vitamins Network

http://www.vitamins.net

Click **Vitamins and Minerals Guide,** which presents the benefits, RDA, best food sources, synergistic nutrients, deficiency symptoms, and negative interactions of each vitamin and mineral.

Vitamins and Minerals

http://www.nal.usda.gov/fnic/etext/000068.html#v&m

This page from The Food and Nutrition Information Center has links to other sites' reputable articles on an array of vitamins and minerals. The FNIC is part of the United States Department of Agriculture (USDA).

Do You Know Your Vitamin ABCs?

http://www.cspinet.org/nah/9_99/vitamin_abc.htm

If you try to keep up with vitamin news, take this tough, 30-question test from Nutrition Action Health Letter to see if your knowledge is current. I'll bet you can't get a perfect score.

Recommended Dietary Intakes

http://www.nal.usda.gov/fnic/dga/rda.pdf

For more than 50 years, nutrition experts have used a set of nutrient and energy (calorie) standards known as the Recommended Dietary Allowances (RDA). Experts are working now to revise these standards. This chart presents the RDA for 15 nutrients plus the new recommendations, called Dietary Reference Intakes (DRI) for five additional nutrients. The chart categorizes recommendations by gender, age, and other specifics. This is a PDF file—you need Acrobat Reader to view it.

Straight Answers About Vitamin and Mineral Supplements

http://www.eatright.org/nfs/nfs66.html

Before you load up on supplements, read this basic advice from The American Dietetic Association.

Start Here: Drug Information Sites

You want to get the scoop on a medication and you don't want to spend your time worrying whether you're getting the right information. All these sites give accurate information in a format that's easy to find and presented in simple, lay person's language.

Personal Drugstore: Dr. Koop

http://www.drkoop.com/hcr/drugstore/

Read news about drugs, participate in chats, and check drug interactions on this authoritative site. A cool feature is the Drug Checker where you type in the drugs you're taking or want to know about. You can read a clear, simply worded information guide on each one, plus check interactions. Includes a directory of pharmacies that can fill your prescriptions online.

DrugDigest.org

http://www.drugdigest.org/

You can look up drugs, vitamins, and herbs; read news, research, and treatment tips; join a discussion group; and ask a pharmacist a private question (see Figure 14.3). This site includes lots of information, and they're not pushing anything.

adam.com

http://www.adam.com/

If you know the medical condition but don't know what drugs to look up, this site can help. Do a search on the condition, and then click **drug leaflets** in the result type box. You end up with the same drug database used by Koop (from Multum Information Services). You might also want to read the news stories related to drugs and your disease.

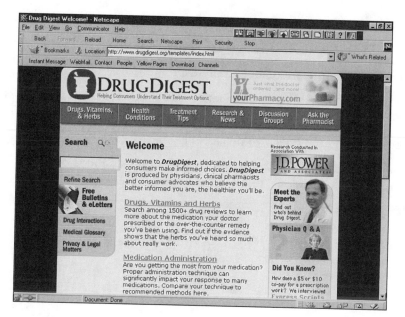

Figure 14.3

DrugDigest helps consumers make informed decisions.

Discovery Health

http://www.discoveryhealth.com

Click **Rx Central** which gives you a variety of medication pages, such as Ask the Pharmacist, Today's Drug News, Recent Articles, Disease-Specific Drugs, Johns Hopkins Drug Commentaries, Drug Basics, and Poison Control. Or click **Alternative Medicine**, and then **Herbal Medicines** to learn about herbs.

iVillage allHealth

http://www.allhealth.com/

Click **drug database** to get the Medications Resource Page, where you can search by medication, browse the database alphabetically, or read articles about over-the-counter medications or the effects of certain drugs on pregnancy.

The Least You Need to Know

➤ You can find extensive information about a prescription medication online.

➤ Buying medications online can be a convenience, but check out the e-pharmacy first.

➤ Herbs are medicines, and they need to be carefully researched.

➤ Drugs, including herbs, can interact with one another or affect a medical condition; get a health professional's recommendation before you medicate.

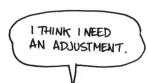

I THINK I NEED AN ADJUSTMENT.

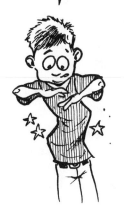

Chapter 15

Alternative/ Complementary Medicine

In This Chapter

➤ Finding and exploring online alternative/complementary medicine resources

➤ Evaluating alternative treatment claims

➤ Spotting and avoiding scams

Alternative medicine is perhaps the most controversial area of health care. Some people believe in it with a religious fervor. Others see the whole movement as a giant hoax. Most of us are somewhere in the middle, looking for therapies and products that hold promise and discarding those that don't. Even experts disagree about how to cleanly divide various alternative methods into "useful" and "useless," so this chapter wriggles out of that job, too.

Here's what this chapter can do: It can point you to sites where you can get good information, and which seem to be more reliable than most. It doesn't endorse or slam any particular therapies here—it just shows you how to explore them if you're so inclined. This chapter gives you some potent tools for recognizing sites that are disseminating accurate information versus those just hyping their own agenda and hoping for a slice of your bank account. You read what the gurus and the skeptics have to say and decide for yourself.

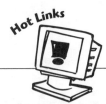

What Is Alternative Medicine?

http://www.healthatoz.com/atoz/centers/alternative/altwhat.asp

"What is complementary and alternative medicine, and why are so many people willing to spend so much time and money on it?" This excellent, unbiased introduction to alternative medicine discusses the differences between alternative and conventional therapies, the major fields of alternative practice, and a comparison of conventional and alternative approaches to five common medical conditions.

What Can You Find?

Alternative medicine, although it's thousands of years old, addresses a need in modern society. It's more personal than the 15-minute appointment and prescription you often get from your physician. It puts you in control of your treatment and lets you participate in your healing, rather than being a passive recipient. Fifty percent of patients in a recent survey said they use some form of alternative medicine. It's a blossoming field.

Alternative medicine is also known as complementary medicine, emphasizing that these different therapies can complement Western medicine and don't have to be at odds with it. Different practitioners use the handles they prefer. A new term is *integrative medicine,* used by health practitioners who combine alternative and Western therapies.

The World Wide Web can quench your thirst for knowledge whether you're interested in acupuncture, chiropractic, homeopathy, hypnotherapy, reflexology, or any of dozens of other practices. The Web has opened up a world of opportunity for learning about any alternative option you could imagine and many you couldn't.

More alternative therapies exist than can possibly be covered in one chapter. This chapter just points you to a few samples of the many alternative therapies that you can explore on the Web, with recommended "go here first" sites.

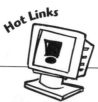

Hot Links

Of Allopaths And Ayurvedics: An Introduction to Systems of Medicine

```
http://healthcentral.com/news/
column_schmalz.cfm?ID=17685&storytype=Column_Schmalzp
```

This article from Rochelle Perrine Schmalz, M.S.L., HealthCentral's medical librarian, describes several philosophies and practices of the art and science of medicine. Learn how allopathic medicine (our modern Western medical system) differs from a selection of Eastern and complementary systems, with a site recommendation for learning more about each one. If you can't stand to type the whole URL, go to `http://healthcentral.com`, click **News**, **Columnists**, **Rochelle Perrine Schmalz**. If the article you want isn't the one that pops up, scroll to the bottom for a list of all of Schmalz's articles.

Acupuncture

Acupuncture, an ancient Chinese healing method, uses tiny needles to stimulate the nerves in skin and muscle to relieve pain and achieve other health benefits.

Alternative Medicine Therapies: Acupuncture

```
http://library.advanced.org/24206/acupuncture.html
```

What does acupuncture accomplish, how does it work, and what does it look like? Find out here, from Alternative Medicine Online, which also has pages on 20 other alternative therapies.

American Academy of Medical Acupuncture

```
http://www.medicalacupuncture.org
```

Medical acupuncture means "acupuncture that has been successfully incorporated into medical or allied health practices in Western countries." Learn about the research and find a physician/acupuncturist at this site.

Ayurvedic Medicine

Ayurveda is a 4,000-year-old Indian method of healing, which believes that each person has an individual "constitution" that can be classified into three dominant types and determines a particular diet and lifestyle to achieve balance.

Ayurveda: Brief Introduction and Guide

http://www.ayurveda.com/info/Ayurintro.htm

This article from The Ayurvedic Institute by Dr. Vasant Lad is maybe the clearest explanation on the Web of what Ayurvedic medicine is, how it works, and how to apply the principles.

Biofeedback

Biofeedback is a treatment technique that trains people to use signals from their own bodies to improve their health. Biofeedback can help you relieve tension and anxiety, or cope with pain. Physical therapists use it to help stroke victims regain movement in paralyzed muscles.

What Is Biofeedback?

http://www.healthy.net/library/articles/biofeedback/biofeedbackwhatis.htm

This article from the U.S. Department of Health and Human Services describes what biofeedback is, how it is used, and how it works.

Chinese Medicine

Chinese medicine is a system for diagnosis, treatment, and wellness with a 23-century track record.

Understanding Chinese Medicine from HealthWorld Online

http://www.healthy.net/clinic/therapy/chinmed/specifics/underst.htm

This information-rich site has articles on many aspects of Chinese medicine: basic principles, history, diagnosis, and how it works.

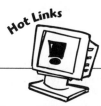

Separating Hype from Hope: Making Sense of Complementary Medicine Research

http://my.webmd.com/topic_summary_article/DMK_ARTICLE_58948

Usually there's no expert consensus on whether or not an alternative treatment works, so it's important for you, the potential user, to understand how to evaluate whatever evidence is presented. This article describes the different kinds of evidence, and how to evaluate complementary-treatment claims.

Chiropractic

Chiropractors adjust and manipulate the musculoskeletal system, especially the spinal column, to alleviate pain and imbalance.

American Chiropractic Association

http://www.amerchiro.org/

Click **About Chiropractic** to learn what chiropractic is and read consumer tips such as how to "pull your weeds, not your back" and how to wear backpacks properly. You can also find a local chiropractor.

Feldenkrais

The Feldenkrais Method improves daily-life function by teaching the neuromuscular system new movement patterns through gentle, precise movements.

About the Feldenkrais Method

http://www.feldenkrais.com

This site from the Feldenkrais Guild of North America not only explains the practice, but also lets you experience it with online lessons especially for computer users.

Macrobiotics

A macrobiotic diet is simple, pure, and balanced, emphasizing whole grains and vegetables and avoiding processed foods.

203

Macrobiotics Online

http://www.macrobiotics.org/

This site from the Kushi Institute, a well-known macrobiotic education center, shares the philosophy of the macrobiotic way of life, disease-recovery case studies, and an assortment of recipes.

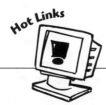

How to Use Alternative and Complementary Medicine

http://my.webmd.com/topic_summary_article/DMK_ARTICLE_58289

This helpful, unbiased article from WebMD, includes research evidence, information on choosing a complementary therapy, a guide to choosing a practitioner. It points out that alternative medicine is not always harmless.

Where's the Science? Fact Versus Fantasy, Opinion, and Anecdote

Many alternative therapies are popular because of opinion, anecdote, and hope. That doesn't mean they don't work, but it doesn't prove they do, either. We're not saying to wait until the research is in before getting a massage or a chiropractic adjustment when you know darn well how good these treatments feel. If your back hurts and your friend felt much better after a Reiki treatment, go ahead and try it out. We're just saying that if you're counting on an alternative treatment to treat a disease or medical condition, realize that testimonials and anecdotes aren't proof.

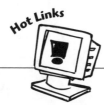

FDA Guide to Choosing Medical Treatments

http://www.fda.gov//oashi/aids/fdaguide.html

How can you tell which alternative treatment might help treat your condition, and which might make you worse (financially and physically)? This site outlines how the FDA evaluates the safety and efficacy of a new treatment, discusses some alternative therapies that are being studied, and provides "TipOffs to RipOffs" for evaluating scam treatments.

I Believe: The Placebo Effect

One reason that testimonials are so popular in ads is that you can always find people who earnestly believe that their psoriasis cleared or their chronic fatigue lifted because of this one product or procedure. So, realize that when you hear about people who got the results you're seeking from an untested treatment, you don't know whether their improvement was actually due to the treatment, or other treatments, or spontaneous remission, or the placebo effect.

The placebo effect occurs when people take some product or undergo some process and experience a benefit because they believe they will. The mind is incredibly potent, and the power of suggestion can achieve what seem to be miraculous results. More than 30 percent of people improve with a treatment that is worthless, just because they believe in it!

"So what, as long as it works?" you might ask. But if someone else got better because of the placebo effect, you don't know whether *your* belief in the treatment will work as powerfully. Besides, if your mind is that strong, why not harness the power of your mind and heal yourself without mailing hefty checks to a placebo provider?

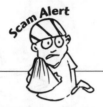

Rally Your Forces

Before you sink money into an alternative treatment that might or might not be useful, check with your doctor, pharmacist, or other health professional. No, they are not in collusion to steer you toward expensive pharmaceuticals or medical treatments. They *are* in collusion to protect your health. If the product you're considering is unwarranted or a scam, they know about it and can head you off before you spend your money. You can also check out a product with the Better Business Bureau and government agencies such as your state's Attorney General, the Federal Trade Commission, the Food and Drug Administration, and, if it's sold through the mail, your Postmaster.

Recognizing Red Flags

The same red flags we've talked about before are waving madly in alternative-medicine scams. Hide your money and be especially wary when you see any of the following "4 Cs":

➤ **Come-ons** Words such as "secret" or "miracle."

➤ **Conspiracy allegations** "The medical establishment/AMA/pharmaceutical companies don't want you to know!"

➤ **Cure-all claims** There is no product or therapy that can cure everything from arthritis to zits.

➤ **CAPITAL LETTERS AND EXCLAMATION POINTS!!!!!!!!!**

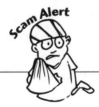

Bunko Squad—Quack, Quack??

http://www.wellweb.com/altern/bunko/bunko.htm

This bunko blaster is from the U.S. Department of Health and Human Services. It's the same information that this chapter emphasizes, but maybe you're more likely to believe it if it comes from a government resource.

Start Here: Best Alternative/Complementary Sites

The following sites are recommended sources of information about alternative/complementary medicine. Many of our "Medical Super Sites" also have good alternative-medicine sections.

HealthWeb's Alternative/Complementary Medicine

http://www.medsch.wisc.edu/chslib/hw/altmed/

This site from HealthWeb and the University of Wisconsin-Madison provides annotated links to numerous alternative treatments: Eastern, Western, manual, herbal, mind/body, and therapies for specific health conditions. It's all here.

Ask NOAH About: Alternative (Complementary) Medicine

http://www.noah.cuny.edu/alternative/alternative.html

This assortment of links to a variety of alternative treatments and approaches from New York Online Access to Health (NOAH) is a good place to start exploring.

WellnessWeb: Alternative/Complementary Medicine

http://www.wellweb.com/AlternativeComplementary_Medicine.htm

This unbiased site includes friendly advice for using complementary therapies for different conditions, with links to other sites and research press releases. Be sure to read the useful overview.

Ask Dr. Weil

http://www.pathfinder.com/drweil/

Andrew Weil, M.D., the father of integrative medicine, answers questions and recommends natural treatments for a variety of ailments. (Although he is greatly respected in the alternative-medicine field, realize that his major sponsor is a supplement retailer, and he recommends supplements widely.)

The National Center for Complementary and Alternative Medicine (NCCAM)

http://nccam.nih.gov

NCCAM, a branch of the National Institutes of Health, conducts and supports research and distributes information on complementary and alternative medicine (CAM). Articles on choosing and using CAM are helpful and trustworthy, although the writing style is a bit stodgy for our taste. Use the Citation Index to research specific therapies and diseases to get abstracts about research findings. (Be careful to narrow your search. A search on "asthma" and "all" CAM therapies yielded more than 2,000 reports, for example.)

Alternative Health News Online

http://www.altmedicine.com/

This is a frequently updated gateway to sites that a group of journalists consider "the most helpful alternative, complementary, and preventive health news pages on the Internet." Learn about Chinese medicine, hypnosis, naturopathic medicine, or any other familiar or unfamiliar alternative therapy. You get news developments, warnings, consumer news, and links.

HealthSCOUT

http://www.healthscout.com

Scroll down to **Directory** and click **Alternative Medicine** for an interesting assortment of articles—both background and news—about 17 different alternative practices, including aromatherapy, biofeedback, Chinese medicine, hypnosis, and polarity therapy.

Alternative Medicine

http://www.healthatoz.com/atoz/centers/alternative/altindex.asp

This is an excellent first stop to get an overview of alternative medicine and an introduction to the most popular therapies (see Figure 15.1), such as acupuncture, aromatherapy, bodywork therapies, chiropractic care, and herbalism.

Figure 15.1

HealthAtoZ offers introductions to several alternative medicine therapies.

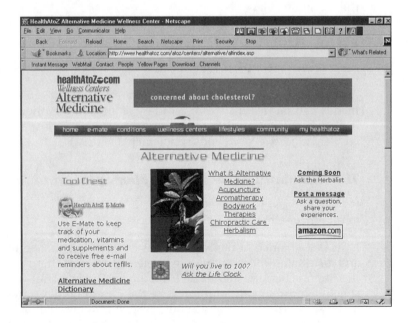

Alternative Medicine Homepage

http://www.pitt.edu/~cbw/altm.html

This popular site from the University of Pittsburgh describes itself as "a jumpstation for sources of information on unconventional, unorthodox, unproven, or alternative, complementary, innovative, and integrative therapies." You can find science-based databases, reviewed sites, and links to alternative treatments for a variety of diseases.

The Least You Need to Know

➤ You can locate information about any kind of alternative or complementary medical treatment on the Web.

➤ Educate yourself about what evidence supports an alternative-medicine claim.

➤ Be wary of sites that use only testimonials to promote a particular treatment.

Part 5
Diseases and Disorders

When you have a disease or other medical disorder, it's easy to fall into feelings of powerlessness and passivity—which can make you sicker. The information you get online can help you out of that cycle. There's nothing so empowering as charging into your doctor's office with your arms full of printouts and a mind full of information and questions. It turns you into an active participant in your medical care—and maybe your physician's cyber-assistant!

This section kick-starts your exploration of some of the medical conditions that are searched for most often on the Web. You learn the most informative and most credible sites for 10 different diseases and disorders—with information in language you can understand without a medical degree.

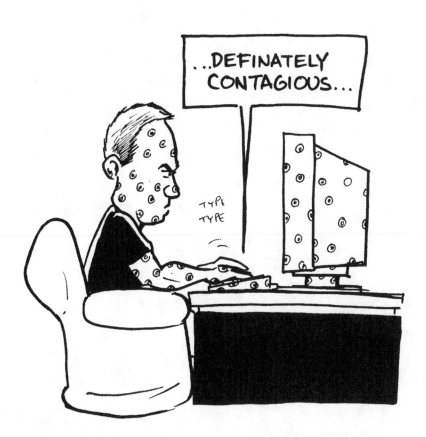

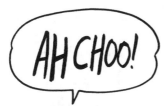

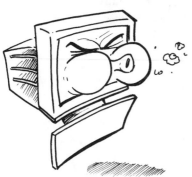

Chapter 16

Allergies and Asthma

In This Chapter

➤ Getting allergy information online

➤ Learning about asthma and how to control it

➤ Helping a child with allergies or asthma

Although allergies and asthma are not the same, allergies might trigger asthma, and many sites cover both conditions. So that's what is done in this chapter.

This chapter introduces you to the sites that can help you manage your allergies or asthma, and offers help for children with these conditions, too.

Allergies

About one in five Americans suffers from an allergy to at least one substance. Allergic reactions can be bothersome—such as sneezing, itchy eyes, or a skin rash—or very serious, even life-threatening—such as impaired breathing.

If you suffer from an allergy to pollen, known as hay fever (also called allergic rhinitis), you have plenty of company. Hay fever affects an estimated 10 percent of Americans (26 million people) and is the reason for 9.2 million office visits to physicians yearly, according to the Centers for Disease Control.

Hay fever is not the only kind of allergy. Other common allergens are mold spores, dust mites, animal dander, feathers, foods, medications, and insect stings, according to the American Academy of Allergy, Asthma, and Immunology. Some—like food and pet allergies—you have to learn to avoid. Others—like the dreaded hay fever—cannot be avoided (unless you move to a region that doesn't have any of your triggers growing), but medications are often effective.

The term *allergy* means that your immune system reacts abnormally to a substance that is usually not harmful. Whatever allergy is making you sneeze, wheeze, or swell, you can learn about it from the World Wide Web.

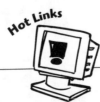

Fast Facts: Frequently Asked Questions (FAQs)

http://www.aaaai.org/public/fastfacts/faq.stm

What are allergies and how do you know if you have them? The American Academy of Allergy, Asthma, and Immunology answers basic questions.

Start Here: Allergy Sites

The following sites give you an introduction to allergies, and then let you delve deeper.

Patient/Public Resource Center

http://www.aaaai.org/public/default.stm

This is the consumer section of the American Academy of Allergy, Asthma, and Immunology site, where you can read articles about many basic topics concerning allergies and asthma.

Allergy Center

http://onhealth.com/ch1/condctr/allergy/item,38757.asp

The Allergy Condition Center from OnHealth in association with the Allergy, Asthma, and Immunology Division at Scripps Clinic, is a detailed patient guide on allergies, including basics, tests, treatment, and resources.

Sniffles & Sneezes

http://www.allergyasthma.com/

This site offers allergy and asthma care and prevention for the family from Louise H. Bethea, M.D., an allergist/immunologist in the North Houston area. Learn about hay fever, insect-sting allergies, latex allergies, exercise-induced asthma, and much more.

Allergy & Asthma Center

http://www.mayohealth.org/mayo/common/htm/allergy.htm

This site from the Mayo Clinic covers every allergy topic you can imagine: hay fever, sinus infections (often mistaken for a cold), food allergies, pet allergies, drug allergies, even latex allergies (see Figure 16.1).

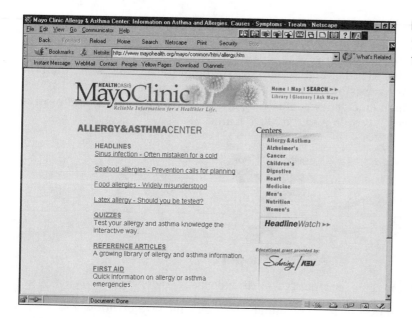

Figure 16.1

The Mayo Clinic covers a variety of allergy topics.

Food Allergies

Food allergies are not common—only about three percent of children and one percent of adults have clinically proven allergic reactions to foods.

Chances are, if a food doesn't "agree" with you, you have an intolerance (which is unpleasant but not dangerous). A true food allergy, however, causes devastating illness and can be deadly, so it's important to learn the difference. Most food allergies are caused by milk, peanuts, other nuts, eggs, fish, shellfish, wheat, soy, or beans.

If you suspect you have a food allergy, call your doctor. While you're waiting for your appointment, avoid those foods and explore the following sites.

Information About Food Allergies

http://www.foodallergy.org/information.html

Get the facts about food allergies from the Food Allergy Network, including which foods cause them, symptoms, and what you can do about them.

Food Allergies: Rare But Risky

`http://vm.cfsan.fda.gov/~dms/wh-alrg1.html`

This is an excellent and detailed article from the FDA about food and food-additive allergies, including the problem of verifying whether a forbidden product is contained in a particular food.

Asthma

Asthma is a chronic respiratory disease that causes a tightening of the chest and difficulty breathing due to inflammation and narrowing of the airways. More than 14 million Americans have asthma—4.8 million are children under the age of 18. Asthma causes 3 million emergency room visits, 500,000 hospitalizations, and nearly 6,000 deaths every year, according to the Mayo Clinic.

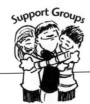

Asthma Support

`http://www.thriveonline.com/health/asthma/connect/index.html`

Find support from ThriveOnline's community, including message boards where people with asthma share stories and medication experiences, parents of asthmatic children share advice, and teens share embarrassments and solutions.

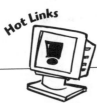

Fast Facts: Famous People with Asthma

`http://www.aaaai.org/public/fastfacts/famous.stm`

Dennis Rodman, Jim "Catfish" Hunter, Liza Minelli, Alice Cooper, John F. Kennedy, Olympic medallists Jackie Joyner-Kersee, Nancy Hogshead, Tom Dolan, Jim Ryun, Kurt Grote, Greg Louganis, and many more—read this surprising list of famous people who had/have asthma, from the American Academy of Allergy, Asthma, and Immunology.

Asthma is a treatable disease that can be managed with medication and self-monitoring. Thanks to recent medical advances, you and your doctor can figure out a combination of medications and procedures (monitoring your breathing and recognizing triggers and warning signs, for example) that keep you (or your child) safe and breathing.

An asthma attack can feel like you're trying to breathe with an elephant standing on your chest. If you don't have asthma, here's an exercise from the Mayo Clinic to show you what it feels like: "Put a straw in your mouth and close your lips tightly around it. Hold your nose. Now exhale. Imagine climbing stairs or trying to sleep."

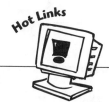

Asthma Management Plan

`http://www.mayohealth.org/mayo/9904/htm/plan.htm`

What should you do in an asthma emergency? What are your personal signs that tell you to seek care quickly? This asthma management plan comes in three zones patterned after traffic lights. Print it out and take it to your doctor to fill out, then keep it handy. You'll need a peak flow meter (`http://www.mayohealth.org/mayo/9904/htm/meter.htm`) to use this plan effectively.

Start Here: Asthma Sites

The allergy sites listed earlier in this chapter have solid information about asthma, as well. Learn more about asthma specifically at the following sites.

Asthma

`http://www.ama-assn.org/insight/spec_con/asthma/asthma.htm`

The asthma site from the American Medical Association has detailed articles about living with asthma, medications, triggers, managing attacks, using inhalers properly, and much more.

Asthma Control

`http://www.mayohealth.org/mayo/9602/htm/asthma.htm`

This superb, comprehensive asthma guide from the Mayo Clinic explains asthma causes, triggers, diagnosis, treatment, and self-management. You'll also find articles about asthma and children, and interactive quizzes. There's more here than your doctor ever told you!

Asthma Center

http://onhealth.com/ch1/condctr/asthma/item,40008.asp

The Asthma Condition Center from OnHealth in association with the Allergy, Asthma, and Immunology Division at Scripps Clinic, is a detailed patient guide on asthma, including basics, diagnosis, monitoring, management, and resources.

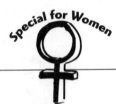

Special for Women

What If You Have Asthma and Are Pregnant?

http://www.ama-assn.org/insight/spec_con/asthma/pregnant.htm

This article from the American Medical Association describes what you should be aware of if you're pregnant and have asthma, what to do, and concerns about medications.

Your Asthma Can Be Controlled: Expect Nothing Less

http://rover.nhlbi.nih.gov/health/public/lung/asthma/asthma.htm

This multi-page guide from the National Asthma Education and Prevention Program of the National Institutes of Health combines helpful information with worksheets that can be printed and filled out to help you understand your asthma better and create a personalized plan.

American Lung Association

http://www.lungusa.org/

Click **Asthma** to see a list of topics: general asthma, adult asthma, and children with asthma. Some sections are written for kids, like the story of Bronkie, the dinosaur with asthma.

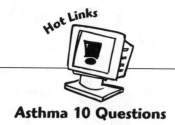

Asthma 10 Questions

http://my.webmd.com/content/article/1660.50014

Are there things I can change in my environment to reduce my risk of attacks? Should I take my medication even if I feel fine? WebMDHealth provides a list of 10 questions to ask your doctor about asthma to help you understand your condition and how to treat it.

Kids and Asthma

Asthma is one of the most common chronic diseases of childhood, according to the American Lung Association, affecting an estimated 4.8 million children under 18 years old. Asthma is the most common cause of school absenteeism due to chronic disease. Unfortunately, children have the steepest recent increases in asthma cases. Second-hand smoke is one major contributor to childhood asthma.

Having to struggle to breathe is terrifying to an adult, so imagine how it must feel to a child.

Fortunately, some excellent sites offer information in words kids can understand (and entertaining enough to hold a child's attention) and wise, comforting advice to parents.

Just for Kids: Coloring Book

http://www.aaaai.org/public/just4kids/coloringbook/default.stm

Kids with allergies or asthma have a site where they can learn, feel relaxed, and enjoy it, thanks to the American Academy of Allergy, Asthma, and Immunology. This coloring book for kids uses superheroes like Dr. Al Lergist, and the "Sneeze and Wheeze Busters" (like Annie Histamine and Buster Bronchodilasaurus) to teach kids about allergies and asthma (see Figure 16.2). Your child clicks the pictures, prints them out, and colors them.

Figure 16.2

The American Academy of Allergy, Asthma, and Immunology's coloring book teaches children about asthma.

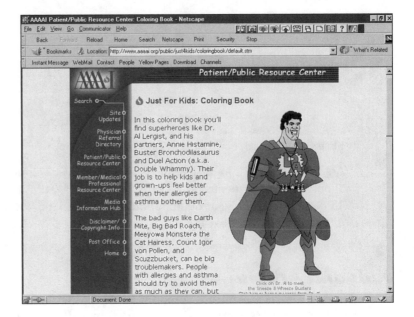

Asthma and Children: Planning for the Next Attack

http://www.mayohealth.org/mayo/9809/htm/asth_prep.htm

As a parent, the worst thing you can do when your child has an asthma attack is panic and fail to act quickly. The Mayo Clinic comes to the rescue with clear, practical, and life-saving information about how to plan ahead for your child's next asthma attack, so that you act efficiently instead of panicking.

The Least You Need to Know

➤ There are many different kinds of allergies, and you can learn about all of them through online resources.

➤ People with asthma can use online resources to understand triggers, proper asthma management, and medications.

➤ Children, as well as their parents, can learn how to manage allergies and asthma from the Internet.

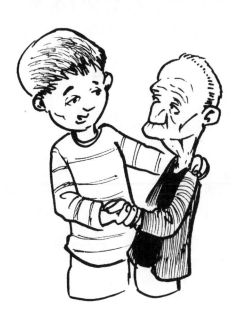

Chapter 17

Alzheimer's Disease

In This Chapter

➤ What Alzheimer's disease is, and how it affects the brain

➤ Recognizing the warning signs of Alzheimer's

➤ Learning how to live with Alzheimer's

Scientists don't know how to prevent or cure Alzheimer's, a progressive disease that affects brain function. If you have a relative or friend with Alzheimer's, you know the heartbreak of watching your loved one lose memory, speech proficiency, and reasoning ability. Learning all you can about the disease won't cure it, but can help you feel less powerless.

This chapter tells you where to find credible information and compassionate support for dealing with Alzheimer's disease.

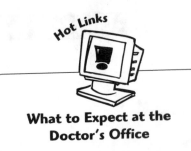

What to Expect at the Doctor's Office

http://www.alzheimers.com/
health_library/diagnosis/
diagnosis_03_doctor.html

What happens when a doctor does a clinical evaluation for Alzheimer's? Find out step-by-step from this helpful site.

Learning About Alzheimer's

Alzheimer's disease is the most common cause of dementia in older people, according to the Alzheimer's Disease Education and Referral (ADEAR) Center (http://www.alzheimers.org/). Dementia means that the way the brain works is disrupted, resulting in loss of intellectual function. Alzheimer's affects the parts of the brain that control thinking, memory, and language.

Alzheimer's is a progressive, degenerative disease that attacks the brain. Nerve cells in the part of the brain responsible for memory and other thought processes degenerate, resulting in impaired thinking, behavior, and memory. Here are some facts from the FDA and the ADEAR Center:

➤ Up to 4 million Americans have Alzheimer's disease.

➤ One in 10 people over age 65 are afflicted with Alzheimer's disease.

➤ Nearly half of all people age 85 and over have Alzheimer's.

➤ Women make up 72 percent of the U.S. population age 85 and older, and nearly one-half of this group has Alzheimer's disease.

➤ Eighty percent of caregivers are women.

➤ The cause of Alzheimer's is unknown, and there is no known cure.

➤ Alzheimer's disease is not a normal part of aging.

Warning Signs

Recognizing early warning signs of Alzheimer's disease is very important. People diagnosed early can benefit from treatments that help while the disease is mild, and can plan for their future.

The following are some early warning signs of Alzheimer's, from the Alzheimer's Association. (For a description of 10 warning signs from the Alzheimer's Association, go to http://www.alz.org/facts/, and click **What are the warning signs?** under **Common Questions**.)

➤ Memory loss that affects job skills

➤ Difficulty performing familiar tasks

➤ Problems with language

➤ Disorientation to time and place

➤ Changes in mood, behavior, and personality

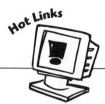

Memory Quiz: How Sharp Are You?

http://www.alzheimers.com/health_library/risk/risk_06_quiz.html

You can't read about Alzheimer's without wondering if you're in the early stages when you forget where you parked your car or can't remember someone's name. This quiz won't tell you if you have Alzheimer's—it's just a memory test that scores you according to the average person in a particular age range.

Stages of Alzheimer's

The FDA recognizes these three broad stages of Alzheimer's disease:

1. Forgetful and aware of it, asking for other people's help or making reminder lists.
2. Severe memory loss (especially about recent events), disorientation, inability to find the right word (dysphasia), and sudden mood changes.
3. Severe confusion and disorientation, sometimes accompanied by hallucinations or delusions, purposeless wandering, incontinence, and neglect of personal hygiene.

The progression of Alzheimer's disease can also be broken down into five or more stages. See **5 Stages of AD** with a list of symptoms and suggestions for what to do at each stage at http://neuro-oas.mgh.harvard.edu/sea/stages.html.

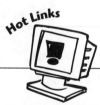

Living with Alzheimer's

http://www.alz.org/taking/Default.htm

This section of the Alzheimer's Association site offers information about what you can expect as the disease progresses, with suggestions on how to live with the changes. See the list of topics at the left. Click **wandering** for information on the Alzheimer's Association's Safe Return program.

Treatment

Two prescription drugs are currently available for the treatment of Alzheimer's: Tacrine (brand name Cognex) and Donepezil (brand Aricept). These drugs improve cognitive functions in some patients in the early stages of the disease, but results vary.

Dozens of medications are being studied, and several show promise. Treatments available today provide only symptomatic relief, but the next generation of treatments might delay onset or slow progression of the disease, according to the Alzheimer's Association.

What Are the Latest Drug Treatments for Alzheimer's Disease?

`http://my.webmd.com/content/dmk/dmk_article_3961785`

This article from WebMDHealth gives an overview of drugs currently approved and therapies showing promise in trials, including nonsteroidal anti-inflammatory drugs, estrogen, and antioxidants.

Alzheimer's Disease Clinical Trials Database

`http://www.alzheimers.org/trials/index.html`

The cure for Alzheimer's will come through research; and this database informs you about clinical trials on Alzheimer's disease and dementia currently in progress in the U.S., how to participate in drug trials, and how to sign up to receive updates on new trials. The Alzheimer's Disease Clinical Trials Database is a joint project of the Food and Drug Administration and the National Institute on Aging (NIA), maintained by the NIA's Alzheimer's Disease Education and Referral (ADEAR) Center.

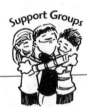

Support Groups

Alzheimer's: A Map for the Journey

`http://www.geocities.com/Heartland/7015/alzheimr.html`

The medical sites give you dependable information, but sometimes you want the human closeness of reading or talking to someone who is going through the same emotions and life changes that you are. This personal site from Sandra Cobb, whose father has Alzheimer's, is not only the story of this family's personal journey, but a wealth of information about how to plan ahead, and connections to other personal sites.

Care Giving

Being a caregiver for a person with Alzheimer's can be a challenging, lonely, frustrating job. The following sites make this easier with information and support.

Alzwell Caregivers Page

http://www.alzwell.com/

Alzwell promises "information, escapes and outlets" for Alzheimer's caregivers. Get caregiver tips, ask questions, tell your story, chat, write on the "anger wall," or read the wrenching postings of others (see Figure 17.1). This is the place to vent and give or get help.

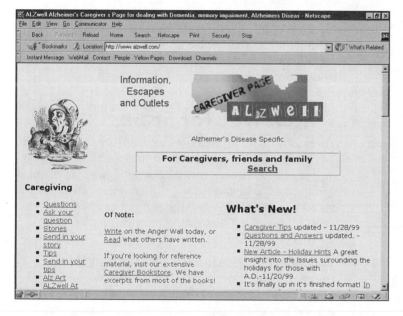

Figure 17.1

Alzwell gives Alzheimer's caregivers support and information.

Understanding and Coping with Problem Behaviors Related to Memory Loss

http://www.vh.org/Welcome/UIHC/UIHCMedDepts/GeriatricEducation/
LearningGuide.html

This helpful guide from the Iowa Geriatric Education Center and Virtual Hospital gives practical ideas for managing an array of problem behaviors. This guide can help you get through all sorts of problems.

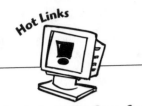

Products to Help Care for Someone with Alzheimer's Disease

http://www.agelessdesign.com/prods.htm

Anti-scalding device, automatic medication dispenser, phone dialer, even a clock radio with a concealed camera—this site offers resources of products that can make the life of a person with Alzheimer's easier or safer.

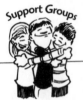

Alzheimer's Support Groups

http://www.alz.org/chapters/

The Alzheimer's Association has 200 chapters across the United States. Click your state to locate a local chapter as a source of information, support, and assistance.

Solutions for Living with Alzheimer's: The Caregiver's Guide to Home Modification

http://www.agelessdesign.com/art-solutions2living.htm

This article from Ageless Design ("Smarter, Safer Living for Seniors") explains how to make your home safe for a person with Alzheimer's. Click **home** to sign up for a free newsletter or leave a question for an expert.

The Elderly Place

http://www.geocities.com/~elderly-place/

This site from social worker Marci Stocks talks about Alzheimer's, with an emphasis on caregiving. Read articles and stories, and get support from the message board and email list.

Watch Out for Scams

There is no cure for Alzheimer's, but there are hundreds of Web sites that claim to have one for sale. Just for fun, I did a search on "Alzheimer's cure" and found 1,900 sites. To be fair, some of them were talking about the fact that a cure for Alzheimer's had not yet been found. But a distressing number of sites sort of claimed to have one.

I say "sort of," because they couched their claims in innuendo and testimonial, so that they weren't coming out and making a false medical claim (there are consequences for that), but they were making you believe it, just the same.

For example, one commercial herb site quotes a ginkgo biloba customer saying, "Thank you for helping me feel like I'm preventing Alzheimer's." (Get it? She "feels like" she's preventing Alzheimer's, but the site—which sells the herb, of course—isn't saying that she is really accomplishing this.)

Trust me, when a cure is discovered, you'll read about it on *all* the reputable medical sites. It won't appear first on a site selling herbs or dietary supplements, or promoting a book. And it certainly won't be hiding on a gaudy, commercial site full of exclamation points, misspellings, and an order form.

When you're looking for information about Alzheimer's, use the Medical Super Sites and the additional sites recommended in this chapter. Don't trust any site that advertises a cure—it just isn't true.

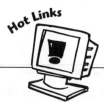

Confronting Alzheimer's: A Guide for Law Enforcement Agencies

`http://www.zarcrom.com/users/alzheimers/cm-index.html`

Marsha Penington created this 40-page manual to help law enforcement personnel better understand the symptoms and problems associated with Alzheimer's and dementia. If you have a family member, friend, or neighbor with Alzheimer's, this guide can help you understand how to be more effective when you want to communicate or have to intervene.

Start Here: Alzheimer's Sites

Now that you know what isn't true, the following sites will tell you what is true.

Alzheimer's Association

`http://www.alz.org/`

The star of Alzheimer's sites, this comprehensive resource is from the Alzheimer's Association. Click **The Facts** for the answers to common questions. Click **Taking Care** for information about living with Alzheimer's. You can also learn about diagnosis, treatment, research, and news stories, or join a local chapter.

Alzheimer's Disease Education and Referral (ADEAR)

`http://www.alzheimers.org/`

The ADEAR Center is from the National Institute on Aging (NIA), one of the National Institutes of Health. It aims to provide "information about Alzheimer's disease, its impact on families and health professionals, and research into possible causes and cures." You can even email or phone to get an answer to your question about Alzheimer's.

Alzheimer's: Few Clues on the Mysteries of Memory

http://www.fda.gov/fdac/features/1998/398_alz.html

This site from *FDA Consumer* is a compassionate yet straightforward explanation of what Alzheimer's disease is, warning signs, stages, and the value of current medications.

Ask NOAH About: Alzheimer's Disease

http://noah.cuny.edu/wellconn/alzheimers.html

This exceptional site is a "Well-Connected" guide to Alzheimer's from Ask NOAH with information on every aspect of Alzheimer's: causes, prevention, symptoms, phases, treatments, and caregiving.

HealthAtoZ.com

http://healthAtoZ.com/

Scroll to **Alzheimer's Disease** under **health topics atoz**. This large site has many valuable articles and message boards. Learn what science understands about causes, risk factors, and treatment. Special articles help you if you're the person with Alzheimer's or the caregiver.

Alzheimer's Disease: Unraveling the Mystery

http://www.mhsource.com/hy/adunravel.html

If you're ready to understand the science, this long article (dated 1995) from the National Institute on Aging gives a scientific explanation of how the disease starts and progresses, the search for causes, research on diagnosis, and more.

The Least You Need to Know

➤ By recognizing the early warning signs, you can help a person with Alzheimer's disease get help and plan for the future.

➤ There is no cure for Alzheimer's, but some treatments might help in the early stages.

➤ Do not fall for scams that promise a cure for Alzheimer's or restoration of memory.

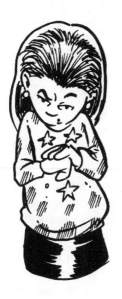

Chapter 18

Arthritis

In This Chapter

➤ Learning about the different forms of arthritis

➤ Exploring ways to manage pain

➤ Learning cautions about unproven treatments

➤ Finding ways to live productively with arthritis

If you're among the 43 million Americans who have arthritis, you're hungry for information about how to relieve your pain and manage your condition. You can learn plenty about arthritis on the Internet, including what causes it, what you can do about it, and ways to live with it. This chapter gives you the most helpful sites for arthritis information.

Arthritis Basics

Arthritis—which literally means joint inflammation—is characterized by pain, swelling, stiffness, and tenderness in the joints. It is a chronic condition, meaning that it doesn't go away.

Consider these facts about the impact of arthritis, from the Arthritis Foundation (`http://www.arthritis.org/resource/fs/arthritis.asp`):

➤ Nearly 43 million Americans have arthritis—one in every six people.

➤ Arthritis is the number one cause of movement limitation in the United States.

➤ Arthritis affects people of all ages, including 285,000 children.

➤ Women make up nearly two-thirds of the people with arthritis.

➤ Nearly 3 million Americans are limited in their daily activities (such as walking, dressing, or bathing) due to arthritis.

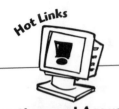

Questions and Answers About Arthritis Pain

http://www.nih.gov/niams/ healthinfo/arthpain.htm

Learn the basics about arthritis pain from the National Institute of Arthritis and Musculoskeletal and Skin Diseases, including causes, treatments, and ways you can minimize pain.

Types

Arthritis is not one disease—it refers to more than 100 different diseases that cause pain, swelling, and limited movement in joints and connective tissue. The following are the most common forms:

➤ **Osteoarthritis** Also known as degenerative joint disease, the most common type of arthritis is characterized by a breakdown of cartilage in the joints.

➤ **Rheumatoid arthritis** This type of chronic arthritis affects joints symmetrically (on both sides of the body) and might also affect the skin, heart, lungs, nerves, blood, eyes, or kidneys. It is an autoimmune disease, unlike osteoarthritis.

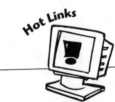

What Is Osteoarthritis?

http://onhealth.com/ch1/condctr/arthritis/item,52756.asp

Osteoarthritis is the most common form of arthritis. What is it, how does it affect joints, what causes it, and how is it treated? This illustrated guide from OnHealth and the Cleveland Clinic's Department of Rheumatic and Immunologic Diseases explains it all.

Other common types include gout, ankylosing spondylitis, juvenile arthritis, and systemic lupus erythematosus. You might not realize that the following conditions are also forms of or related to arthritis: bursitis, tendinitis and myofascial pain, carpal tunnel syndrome, and fibromyalgia.

Learn more about these and other common types and get a brief overview of arthritis from the following sites.

Common Forms of Arthritis Diseases

`http://www.arthritis.org/resource/fs/common_forms.asp`

This site from the Arthritis Foundation explains the different types of arthritis: osteoarthritis, rheumatoid arthritis, gout, ankylosing spondylitis, juvenile arthritis, systemic lupus erythematosus, and other related conditions that affect the joints.

Types of Arthritis

`http://www.arthritis.ca/pages/introduction/`

The Arthritis Society of Canada discusses 19 types of arthritis, with general information, diagnosis, signs and symptoms, risk factors, and treatments for each one.

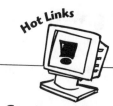

Getting a Grip on Rheumatoid Arthritis

`http://www.arthritis.org/resource/RAcampaign/`

This public information campaign from the Arthritis Foundation presents a series of fact sheets about rheumatoid arthritis, including how it differs from osteoarthritis.

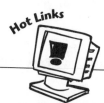

Tell Me More About Juvenile Arthritis

`http://www.arthritis.org/ajao/tellmemore/index.asp`

Juvenile arthritis strikes children ages 15 or younger. About 285,000 children in the United States have a form of juvenile arthritis, the most common type being juvenile rheumatoid arthritis. Learn more about juvenile arthritis from this site from the Arthritis Foundation.

Living with Arthritis

In addition to the medications that your physician prescribes, some lifestyle changes—such as diet and exercise—can help you stay mobile and sometimes decrease the inflammation.

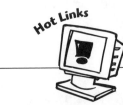

Managing Daily Activities

http://www.arthritis.ca/pages/dailyactivities/

Wind rubber bands around the wide part of a doorknob—with the increased traction, you won't have to grip as hard. Loop pieces of cord through or around the handles of drawers and cupboard doors—then insert your arm to open them, rather than using your wrists and fingers. Click **20 Solutions for Real-World Problems** for these and many other practical tips from the Arthritis Society of Canada.

Diet

Although diet cannot cause or cure arthritis, diet and weight control influence some forms of arthritis, and can help you manage the pain, inflammation, and loss of mobility. The following Web site can help.

Diet

http://www.orthop.washington.edu/Bone%20and%20Joint%20Sources/
xzzzczzz1_2.html

This guide from the University of Washington gives tips for a healthy diet, sensible advice for weight management, and what connections research has found between diet and different forms of arthritis.

Exercise

When your joints ache, the last thing you want to do is exercise, but range-of-motion and stretching exercises are important for joint movement, relief of stiffness, and flexibility.

Exercise and Arthritis Fact Sheet

http://www.arthritis.org/resource/fs/exercise.asp

The Arthritis Foundation offers a number of exercise programs. This fact sheet describes them. Click **local office** to find out what programs your local chapter offers.

Joint Exercises for Arthritis

http://www.arthritis.ca/pages/exercise/

This article explains the importance of exercise for joint mobility. Click **Joint Exercises for Arthritis**, **Select an Exercise** for a variety of animated exercises for different joints (see Figure 18.1). Bookmark this site and return to it often.

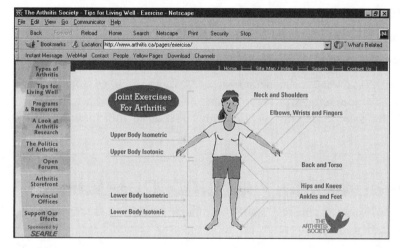

Figure 18.1

The Arthritis Society of Canada presents exercises for arthritic joints.

Exercises and Arthritis

http://www.orthop.washington.edu/Bone%20and%20Joint%20Sources/
xzzzezzz1_2.html

Don't let the ridiculously long URL discourage you from viewing this exceptional site from the University of Washington. Learn not only how exercise helps arthritis, but also what kinds to do and how to do them effectively, with video clips.

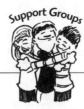

Arthritis Support Groups

The following are some of the message boards, newsgroups, and chats where you can exchange stories, opinions, and questions about arthritis:

➤ `http://www.seniornet.org:8080/cgi-bin/WebX?13@^11640@.ee6ee9b`
SeniorNet Arthritis message boards

➤ `http://www.arthritis.ca/living/wwwboard/wwwboard.html` Arthritis
Society message boards

➤ `news:alt.support.arthritis` Arthritis newsgroup

➤ `news:misc.health.arthritis` Arthritis newsgroup

➤ `http://www.ArthritisWebSite.com/Community/` Chats, message board,
and the chance to nominate your favorite "arthritis warrior": "those folks
who live with the pain of arthritis everyday but put it aside and do wonderful things."

Don't Be Fooled: Avoiding Arthritis Quackery

An arthritis remedy is considered "proven" when in repeated, controlled scientific tests, it reduces pain and swelling, improves functioning, and is safe.

An "unproven" remedy hasn't passed these tests, which means it might or might not work, and even if it works for one person, it might not work for another. This gets even more complicated because arthritis symptoms can go into remission naturally, and you might give a new remedy credit for your improvement when it's just coincidence.

Many people with arthritis feel driven to try unproven remedies—to the tune of $10 billion a year. But even if the unproven remedy is harmless, it can become harmful if you use it instead of getting treatment from a knowledgeable physician, warns the Arthritis Foundation.

The FDA lists fraudulent arthritis products as one of the top health frauds. These fraudulent products include copper bracelets, Chinese herbal remedies, large doses of vitamins, and snake or bee venom (see the FDA Backgrounder at `http://www.fda.gov/opacom/backgrounders/tophealt.html`). Other unproven remedies include mussel extract, desiccated liver pills, shark cartilage, and honey and vinegar mixtures.

Learn more about unproven remedies and frauds, and how to recognize them, from the following sites.

Unproven Remedies Fact Sheet

http://www.arthritis.org/resource/fs/
unproven.asp

This article from the Arthritis Foundation discusses unproven remedies and how to recognize them, including a helpful checklist under "How Can People Determine If A Remedy Is Unproven?"

Bunko Squad—Quack, Quack??

http://www.wellweb.com/altern/bunko/bunko.htm

Quackery is "the promotion of a medical remedy that doesn't work or hasn't been proven to work"—in other words, fraud. This article from the U.S. Department of Health and Human Services warns you about quackery and tells you how you can protect yourself.

Complementary Therapies

http://www.arthritis.ca/pages/
alt&comtherapies/

The Arthritis Society in Canada discusses various unproven, complementary therapies that hold promise and others that are totally unsubstantiated by scientific studies.

Start Here: Arthritis Sites

When you're ready to get past the basics, the following sites provide an extensive education about arthritis.

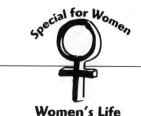

Women's Life

http://www.ArthritisWebSite.
com/Living/Women/

ArthritisWebSite.com examines the special concerns faced by women with arthritis, such as the emotional and physical issues of intimacy, and how pregnancy will affect arthritis.

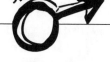

Men's Life

http://www.ArthritisWebSite.
com/Living/men/

ArthritisWebSite.com examines the special concerns faced by men who have or live with someone with arthritis, such as sexual issues and "dos and don'ts for making life with your arthritic loved one less thorny."

Coping with Arthritis in Its Many Forms

http://www.fda.gov/fdac/features/296_art.html

This excellent article from *FDA Consumer* explains what arthritis is, what causes it, the major types, FDA-approved drugs that relieve inflammation and pain and reduce joint damage, the importance of exercise, and how to avoid fraud.

Arthritis Foundation

http://www.arthritis.org/

"The mission of the Arthritis Foundation is to support research to find the cure for and prevention of arthritis and to improve the quality of life for those affected by arthritis." Select **Publications** under "Featured:" for the **Resource Room** for online brochures and fact sheets. The Arthritis Foundation also offers local programs and live support groups.

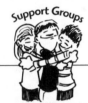

Rheumatology Electronic Communication

http://www.medlib.iupui.edu/
hw/rheuma/listserv.html

This site from HealthWeb offers a collection of listservs and newsgroups addressing arthritis, lupus, fibromyalgia, and more.

The Arthritis Society

http://www.arthritis.ca/home.html

The Arthritis Society of Canada presents a wealth of information about 19 types of arthritis, research, complementary treatments, and tips for living well with arthritis.

HealthAtoZ.com

http://healthAtoZ.com/

Click **arthritis** under **diseases & conditions** for a selection of articles on every aspect of arthritis, including several types of arthritis, effective medications, arthritis and kids, and self-care strategies.

Arthritis Center

http://onhealth.com/ch1/condctr/arthritis/item,51626.asp

OnHealth's Arthritis Medical Center, in association with the Cleveland Clinic's Department of Rheumatic and Immunologic Diseases, presents a variety of in-depth guides to arthritis, covering both the basics and 17 individual disorders.

ArthritisWebSite

http://www.ArthritisWebSite.com/

ArthritisWebSite.com and ArthritisNet.com have merged to bring you the ArthritisWebSite, with a primary focus on "the whole person, not just the disease." Get information with a sense of community (see Figure 18.2).

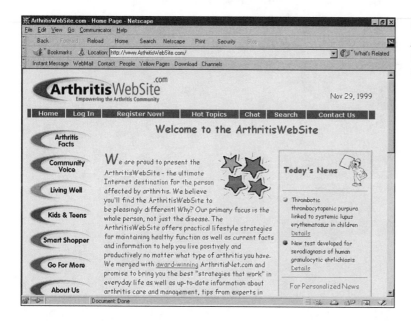

Figure 18.2

ArthritisWebSite merges information and community.

MedlinePlus Arthritis

http://www.nlm.nih.gov/medlineplus/arthritis.html

This site from the National Library of Medicine offers myriad links to other reputable medical and government sites on arthritis, including specific conditions and treatments.

The Least You Need to Know

➤ Arthritis is actually more than 100 diseases that cause joint pain and inflammation.

➤ You can manage the impact of arthritis on your life with medications, diet, exercise, and modifying daily activities.

➤ Avoid spending money on unproven therapies.

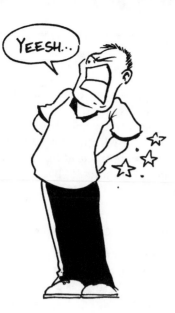

Chapter 19

Back Pain

In This Chapter

➤ Learning how back injuries happen

➤ Preventing overuse back injuries

➤ Managing chronic pain

About 80 to 90 percent of Americans will experience severe back pain at some time in their lives through repetitive-stress injuries (doing an action over and over that the back doesn't like) or acute injuries (getting hurt suddenly due to an accident or fall). Most back pain is felt in the lower back.

This chapter shows you how to find information about the anatomy of your back, how it works, and how it gets injured, with prevention and treatment options.

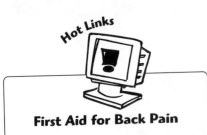

Hot Links

First Aid for Back Pain

http://www.texasback.com/html
/first_aid_for_back_pain.html

"Take A-I-M: Anti-Inflammatories, Ice Massage, and Movement" is the advice of the Texas Back Institute in Plano, Texas. This site tells you exactly what to do and when to do it.

Back Basics

Back pain is the number one work-related medical problem in the United States and the second most common cause of missed workdays. Although roughly 90 percent of people recover within 12 weeks, back injuries that don't recover are the leading cause of disability between the ages of 19 and 45. Back pain is more likely to occur during the productive ages of 30 to 50.

Back pain usually happens in one of two ways:

➤ **Acute**   An acute or traumatic back injury comes from a sudden, unpredictable accident that damages the back, such as a fall or other impact.

➤ **Repetitive stress**   A small action that stresses the back over and over again can lead to injury. Most back injuries are from repetitive stress and, therefore, preventable. These are also called *overuse injuries.*

Most back injuries are self-limited, meaning that they heal on their own. Some injuries, however, can lead to chronic pain (constant or recurring pain that lasts more than six months) and disability.

The following sites teach you the basics about how your back works, and what is happening when it hurts.

Understanding Back Pain

http://www.lowbackpain.com/pain.html

This site from Arnold J. Weil, M.D., is devoted to helping you understand low back pain. Click the **anatomy** pages to read illustrated descriptions of the vertebral column; spinal cord, discs, and nerves; and back muscles.

All About Low Back Pain

http://www.drkoop.com/conditions/Low_Back_Pain/page_48_236.asp

This overview explains briefly how low back pain happens and the anatomy of the spine.

Patient Education

http://www.aaos.org/wordhtml/pat_educ/lowback.htm

This online brochure on the causes and treatments of low back pain is from the American Academy of Orthopaedic Surgeons.

What to Do When Your Back Is in Pain

http://www.fda.gov/fdac/features/1998/298_back.html

This article from *FDA Consumer* discusses back-pain causes, management, exercise, surgery, and acupuncture.

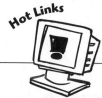

Hot Links

1998 Labor Day CheckList: How to Avoid Low Back Injuries in the Workplace

http://www.acoem.org/whatsnew/98ldchck.htm

Don't wait for Labor Day to take time to use this checklist to review your workplace for health and safety risks. This guide from the American College of Occupational and Environmental Medicine recommends preventive measures for both employers and employees to avoid low back injuries.

Preventing Overuse Injuries

Most back injuries are caused not by a sudden trauma, but by overuse—repetitive stress to the back, either through simple actions done over and over again, or by poor body alignment.

Unlike acute traumatic injury—which you can't anticipate and usually can't prevent—repetitive-stress back injury is completely preventable. It involves postural awareness and avoiding doing activities that repetitively stress the back. Here are some tips:

➤ Keep your spine neutral—neither rounded nor arched.

➤ Keep your chest lifted, abdominals pulled in.

➤ Use your thighs—not your back—to bend and lift.

➤ Avoid repetitive motions where you twist, bend, lift, and reach—especially activities that involve doing two of these at a time.

➤ Stay physically active, and include exercises that strengthen the back and the abdominals.

Posture and Body Mechanics

Many overuse injuries happen on the job, but you might also be stressing your back with daily life activities that make you bend over or twist. Figure out ways to change them by paying attention to your posture and body mechanics (the way you move).

Learning to keep your spine neutral (neither arched nor rounded) and adjusting your daily living activities can help you avoid repetitive-stress injury to your back. You might not be aware of how often you are habitually rounding, arching, or twisting your back.

Do you slump over the sink when you brush your teeth? Try brushing your teeth in the shower so you can stand up straight without making a mess. Do you habitually twist to reach for the phone on your desk? Move the phone so that it's right in front of you. Enlist the help of a family member or co-worker to help you notice ways that you stress your back.

The following sites give you more information about how to protect your back through posture and body mechanics.

Back Up! Guide to a Healthy Back

http://www.fitnesslink.com/exercise/backup.shtml

This excerpt from *Joan Price Says, Yes, You CAN Get in Shape!* (http://www. fitnesslink.com/joanprice/#book) gives you tips for strengthening your back (and appearing slimmer!) through postural alignment. Learn what actions are likely to cause back injury and what to do instead.

Healthy Back Tips

http://www.texasback.com/html/healthy_back_tips.html

Don't sleep on your stomach. Stop smoking (because it reduces the blood supply to the back, which might affect the elasticity of discs and encourage disc degeneration). These and other back care tips are from the book *Treat Your Back Without Surgery* by Stephen Hochschuler, M.D., and Bob Reznik.

Posture for a Healthy Back

http://www4.ccf.org/health/health-info/docs/0300/0359.HTM

"Good posture involves training your body to stand, walk, sit, and lie in positions where the least strain is placed on supporting muscles and ligaments during movement or weight-bearing activities." This illustrated Cleveland Clinic article describes healthy back posture for standing, sitting, driving, and sleeping.

Working Backs

http://www.aomc.org/wkingbacks.html

This superb guide from the Arnot Odgen Medical Center gives detailed instructions for safe techniques of lifting (including lifting another person), sitting, driving, traveling, and even the best ways to protect your back when lifting, bathing, and carrying your baby.

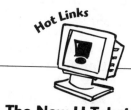

Hot Links

The New LI Teknique

http://www.fitnesslink.com/joanprice/litek.htm

Yes, I'm promoting my own aerobic workout video here, but for a good reason: LI Teknique was designed to strengthen and protect the back. Chiropractors and physical therapists endorse it, and one spine surgeon gives *The New LI Teknique* videotape to his recovering patients. This workout teaches you to stabilize your back while you burn fat aerobically, condition the heart and lungs, strengthen and tone the thighs and buttocks, *and* work the abdominals at the same time! (*LI* is a Chinese character meaning physical strength.)

Exercise

Besides good posture, the single best gift you can give your back is exercise. Stretching, aerobics, and strength training are all important for a healthy back.

Be sure to include abdominal exercises in your back-strengthening program. Weak abdominal muscles let your belly sag, and the extra weight pulls on your back.

The following sites help you design an exercise program that your back will love.

Back Exercises

http://www.fitnesslink.com/exercise/back.shtml

Strengthening your back muscles can help you prevent injury. FitnessLink explains how by describing a variety of strength-training exercises for the major back muscles.

Relieving Low Back Pain with Exercise

`http://www.physsportsmed.com/issues/1997/08aug/shiplepa.htm`

This "Patient Adviser" by Brian Shiple, D.O., published in *The Physician and Sportsmedicine*, describes and illustrates aerobic and back-strengthening exercises and stretches that benefit people with low back pain.

Fitness Prescription for Low Back Pain

`http://healthwatch.medscape.com/`

You have to be a registered member to access this article, but registering is free and painless. Type **"Fitness Prescription for Low Back Pain"** (yes, you need the quotation marks) in the Quick Search box. This article from CBS *HealthWatch* by Medscape describes the FitScriptTM exercise program, consisting of a warm-up, stretching, strength training, aerobic conditioning, and a cooldown, to help manage low back pain. Most strength-training exercises are done in a chair or holding onto a chair.

Extend Yourself for Low Back Pain Relief

`http://www.physsportsmed.com/issues/1997/01jan/back_pa.htm`

This "Patient Adviser" by Louis Kuritzky, M.D., with Jacqueline White, published in *The Physician and Sportsmedicine*, explains the importance of back-extension exercises and shows you how to do them.

Lower-Back Exercises

`http://www.fda.gov/fdac/features/1998/298_exer.html`

This site from *FDA Consumer* and the National Capital YMCA of Washington, D.C., uses animated illustrations to show how to perform exercises that help the lower back (see Figure 19.1).

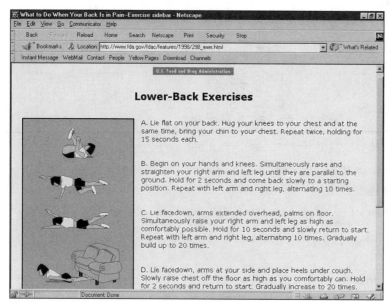

Figure 19.1

Learn four lower-back strengtheners from this site from FDA Consumer and the National Capital YMCA.

Acute Injuries

You rise out of your chair for a moment to talk to someone across the table. You don't realize that a co-worker has come up behind you and pulled your chair out of the way. You start to sit down—on the chair you think is there—and crash to the floor, tailbone first.

You hurt your back suddenly and devastatingly with an acute injury through no fault of your own. Most acute injuries heal, but some—depending on type and severity—become lifelong and life-altering challenges.

Get medical help immediately after an acute injury. You can't tell on your own how severe the injury is, so don't just go home and hope it will go away.

Follow these guidelines for using ice:

➤ Apply ice immediately after the injury, and continue using it for 10–15 minutes every hour to combat swelling.

➤ Do not apply ice directly to the skin. Use a thin towel between your skin and the ice.

➤ Freeze water in a Styrofoam cup. To use the ice, peel away the upper part of the cup and rub.

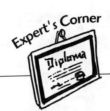

When to See a Doctor

http://www.texasback.com/html/when_to_see_a_doctor.html

If you experience any of the following, you should consider seeing a spine specialist, according to the Texas Back Institute:

➤ The sudden onset of back or neck pain following strenuous activity.

➤ Your back or neck pain has lingered for three weeks or more and you are not improving.

➤ You have pain down the back of your leg.

If you experience any of the following, you should consider it an emergency. See a physician immediately or go to the nearest hospital emergency room.

➤ You begin to drag a leg or foot.

➤ You lose feeling in your arm or hand.

➤ You have loss of bowel or bladder control.

Texas Back Institute spine specialists include chiropractors, physiatrists, and spine surgeons, as well as physicians who specialize in occupational and sports medicine.

Treatment

You have a back injury—what should you do? Bed rest used to be prescribed, but now studies are showing that the sooner you get up and get active, the better you do.

There are myriad treatment options, and the following sites (as well as the "start here" sites at the end of the chapter) help you learn more about them. Be sure to discuss your options and your choices with your physician, and don't omit telling him or her about any alternative treatments you're trying or planning to try.

Realize that whatever the medical prognosis, you can make your recovery go better or worse with your attitude and emotions. Finding online support can help lighten your spirits and give you motivation to work at your healing.

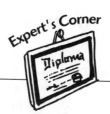

Back Moves

"When your back hurts, try to keep it moving. Particularly avoid prolonged sitting. Get up and stretch or use a lumbar support, preferably one that keeps your back moving."

—Rowland G. Hazard, M.D., Associate Professor of Orthopaedics and Rehabilitation, University of Vermont

Acute Low Back Pain

http://www.quackwatch.com/03HealthPromotion/lbp.html

Learn what treatments are warranted at what stage from this article on QuackWatch by Mark Rosenthal, M.D., assistant professor of orthopaedic surgery at the University of Maryland School of Medicine.

Treatment and Management

http://www.drkoop.com/conditions/Low_Back_Pain/page_48_429.asp

This article gives an overview of ways to treat low back pain, including physical therapy, bracing, medications, injections, surgery, and exercise.

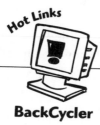

BackCycler

http://www.backcycler.com/

You get more than lumbar support from this air pillow that slowly inflates and deflates, keeping your spine in motion while you're sitting, with you controlling the amount of pressure. Many steps beyond a back massager, this device actually moves the spine and shifts the pattern of stress. Learn more about it at this site.

Acute Low Back Problems in Adults

`http://www.ahcpr.gov/consumer/`

Click **Understanding Acute Low Back Problems, No. 14** under **Consumer Versions of Clinical Practice Guidelines by Condition**. Then click **view** at **Table of Contents**. This patient guide from the Agency for Health Care Policy and Research has information about many topics related to low-back problems, including illustrations and fill-in-the-blanks questions you should answer and take to your doctor.

Three Therapies for Aching Backs

`http://onhealth.com/ch1/in-depth/item/item,47092_1_1.asp`

OnHealth explores three alternative therapies for back pain—acupuncture, chiropractic, and yoga—in this report. Learn what experts in the field say about how, why, and when these complementary therapies can be helpful.

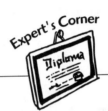

Expert's Corner

Ten Questions to Ask Your Doctor About Back Pain

`http://my.webmd.com/content/article/1661.50014`

WebMDHealth recommends that you print out these 10 questions to take to your next doctor's visit, and take notes on his or her answers:

1. What's causing my back pain?
2. How serious is my condition?
3. Are there activities I should temporarily or permanently avoid?
4. Could my work station be affecting my back pain?
5. What treatment options should I consider?
6. How long should I take medication or do special exercises?
7. How long will it take before I notice results?
8. When can I return to my normal routine?
9. Is there anything else I can do to aid my recovery?
10. What can I do to prevent back pain from persisting or returning?

Chronic Pain

Does your back pain pervade every part of your life? Are your activities limited? Are you angry or depressed because of your pain?

If you suffer from chronic back pain, realize that you can still manage your life and your attitude, with help. The following online resources provide advice and support.

Fighting Back

`http://homepages.primex.co.uk/~backtalk/`

Fighting Back is a branch of BackCare, based in Romford, Essex, England, providing "support, contact, and information service for those with ALL back problems." Learn about pain-management options for chronic pain, including alternative methods. Click **Our Favourite Links** for links to other chronic-pain and treatment Web sites.

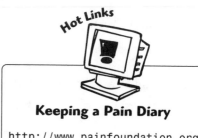

Keeping a Pain Diary

`http://www.painfoundation.org/keeping_a_pain_diary.htm`

This site from the American Pain Foundation teaches you how to keep a pain diary to share with your health-care provider.

American Chronic Pain Association

`http://www.theacpa.org/`

The American Chronic Pain Association "supports self-help groups which teach positive ways to deal with chronic pain." Click **What We Have Learned** for insights about living with chronic pain (see Figure 19.2).

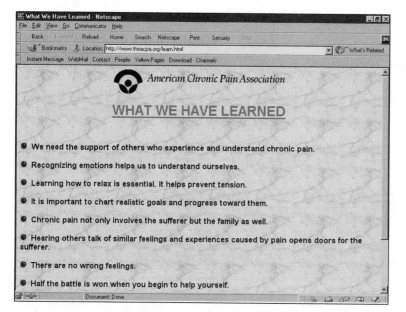

Figure 19.2

Learn insights from the American Chronic Pain Association about living with chronic pain.

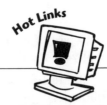

From Patient to Person

`http://www.theacpa.org/steps.html`

These **Ten Steps For Moving From Patient To Person** from the American Chronic Pain Association help you move from a patient whose pain controls your life to a person taking charge of your life through action and attitude adjustment.

Start Here: Back Pain Info Sites

When you're ready to get past the basics, the following sites go into detail about all areas of back pain, from anatomy to symptoms to treatments.

A Patient's Guide to Low Back Pain

`http://www.sechrest.com/mmg/back/backpain.html`

This detailed guide from the Medical Multimedia Group explains the anatomy of the back (with illustrations), causes of different types of injuries, how your physician will diagnose your injury, and an overview of treatments.

Low Back Pain

`http://www.drkoop.com/conditions/low_back_pain/index.asp`

Read news and feature articles about back pain, and join drkoop.com's back-pain chats and message boards.

The Least You Need to Know

➤ More than 80 percent of us are likely to experience severe back pain at some time in our lives.

➤ You can prevent overuse back injuries with posture, body mechanics, and exercise.

➤ You can educate yourself online about treatments for acute injuries.

➤ The Internet provides information and support for chronic pain.

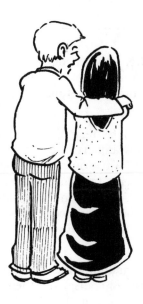

Chapter 20

Cancer

In This Chapter

➤ Finding the best online cancer resources

➤ Learning about different types of cancers

➤ Protecting yourself against scams

➤ Finding support online

Cancer is the most searched-for disease on the Internet. Do a search for "cancer," and you'll find 1.5 million sites. The information (and misinformation) that abounds on the Web is so vast that all this chapter can do is point you to some major resources and give you tips for exploring on your own. After you've educated yourself and you're ready to narrow your focus, you'll find that no matter how specialized your interest, you'll find riches to mine on the Web. This chapter helps you do it, and points you to some of the best general cancer resources and sites for specific cancers.

What Can You Find?

The World Wide Web offers major sites about cancerthat teach you about prevention, risk factors, screening, and explanations of different types of cancer. If you or a loved one has been diagnosed with cancer, you can use the Web to expand your understanding of this disease, how it progresses, and your treatment options. You'll find more sites than you can visit for every type of cancer, no matter how rare, and resources on related topics. Whether you want to learn the basics of how cancer affects cells, the effectiveness of a new treatment, or alternative therapies, online resources give you virtual libraries of reading material. You can learn about and enroll in clinical trials. You can also find incredible support from Internet mailing lists, newsgroups, and chats.

Now the caveat: Beware, beware, beware. Unless you stick to the major sites, much of the information you find can be inaccurate. Recently, researchers from the University of Michigan Health System did an Internet search for information on Ewing's sarcoma, a rare form of malignant bone cancer, and analyzed a sampling of the hits. Nearly half of the 400 Web pages they reviewed contained treatment information that hadn't been medically validated (peer reviewed). About six percent gave inaccurate information, and many more were misleading. The researchers also got hundreds of dead ends, bad links, and pages with no medical information.

So, what can you do to be sure you're getting good information? Stick to the major, most reputable cancer sites (they're listed in this chapter, of course) and their reviewed links. Avoid sliding down the slippery slopes of homegrown sites for your medical information—with a few marvelous exceptions that you see in this chapter.

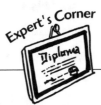

Expert's Corner

"While there are many informative sites about cancer on the Internet, there is also a good deal of unsubstantiated or outdated information online. It is tragic to see patients' survival or quality of life compromised by ill-informed decisions based on misinformation that they have gotten off of the Internet."

—Ted Gansler, M.D., director of health content for the American Cancer Society (http://www.cancer.org)

Treatment Options

This is where the Internet shines. Your doctor will be impressed when you come into the office already knowledgeable about the treatments for your kind of cancer. (To avoid intimidation, though, don't carry in more than three pounds of printouts.) The sites listed as "Start Here" are your gateways to reputable information about medically approved treatments, and if your doc is Internet savvy, he or she can recommend others.

If you want to explore alternative treatments, you have to be especially careful. Yes, some hold promise, but this area is also where the scams, half-truths, unproven therapies, and depositories of wishful thinking reside. The following sites keep you on the safe side of cancer alternative treatments.

Center for Alternative Medicine Research in Cancer

`http://www.sph.uth.tmc.edu/utcam/default.htm`

This site, from the Center for Alternative Medicine Research (UT-CAM) at the University of Texas/Houston Health Science Center, is dedicated to "investigating the effectiveness of complementary/alternative therapies used for cancer prevention and control" (see Figure 20.1). Click **Reviews of Therapies** to see what research has been done on those therapies you've been hearing about, such as garlic, shark cartilage, and a macrobiotic diet. This site is not easy reading, but it's useful and guaranteed to be legit.

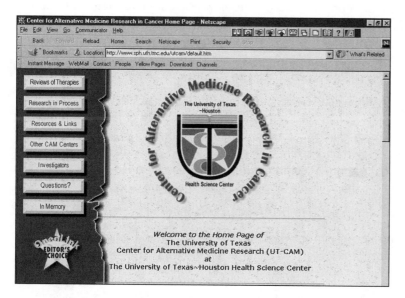

Figure 20.1

The Center for Alternative Medicine Research in Cancer investigates the effectiveness of alternative cancer therapies.

A Special Message for Cancer Patients Seeking "Alternative" Treatments

`http://www.quackwatch.com/00AboutQuackwatch/altseek.html`

Quackwatch, the major watchdog site, has a special letter to cancer patients and dozens of pages about specific quack treatments. Be sure to click **Questionable Cancer Therapies**. This site is always in progress, with articles being added constantly, and Quackwatch lists the reports that aren't quite ready, as well as those that are online. Be patient if the one you want is still in progress.

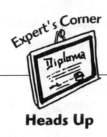

Heads Up

Be careful when viewing these types of sites, warns The American Cancer Society (`http://www.cancer.org`):

➤ Sites that are selling a product—Some sites have accurate information about chemotherapy drugs and other products that may be very useful to people with certain types of cancer. But, it is still important to ask your health care providers whether these treatments are relevant to your type and stage of cancer. Other sites promote products with no proven benefit at all.

➤ Sites provided by individual cancer survivors—Though these sites often provide valuable support and some also provide accurate and objective information, view them with caution. Some survivor's sites contain information overly influenced by their personal experience with a particular type of treatment, which may not accurately reflect whether the treatment is right for you or even for the majority of people with that type of cancer.

➤ Sites that contain information not reviewed by a medical professional.

➤ Sites that are no longer current—With all of the recent and ongoing developments in cancer, it is important to have the most up-to-date information possible.

➤ Sites that are maintained by an unfamiliar organization—Go to the most reputable organizations for accurate information.

The American Cancer Society advises you to share and validate any information gathered from the Internet with a trusted health care provider.

Support

Support groups for cancer abound, and for very good reason. People living with cancer—and the people who love them—need the compassion, information, story sharing, question exchange, and emotion venting that support groups provide.

Psychosocial Support and Personal Experiences

http://www.oncolink.upenn.edu/psychosocial/

This site from OncoLink at the University of Pennsylvania provides many support resources: books, art, and articles about sexuality, coping with cancer, coping with loss and grief, end-of-life issues, spirituality, pain management, and much more.

Y-ME National Breast Cancer Hotline

http://www.y-me.org/

Women with breast cancer and their families and friends will find a national hotline, open door groups, early detection workshops, and many local chapters.

Gillette Women's Cancer Connection

http://www.gillettecancerconnect.org/

This site from Gillette offers resources, advice, and compassionate guidance to help a woman with breast or gynecological cancer, as well as the people who love her.

Share the Hope & Humor

http://www.cancer.med.umich.edu/share/1share.htm

This cancer-support site from the Comprehensive Cancer Center of the University of Michigan Health System delivers warm, compassionate writings and photography from cancer survivors. You'll find poems, short stories, inspirational quotes and humor, and even a song.

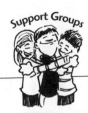

Cancer Support Groups

An average of one in four people who go online to search for information on diseases join an online support group. Here are some places to find cancer newsgroups, message boards, and mailing lists:

➤ `alt.support.cancer` This is a newsgroup for emotional and medical support.

➤ `sci.med.diseases.cancer` This newsgroup offers discussion and information on all types of cancer.

➤ `http://www.acor.org/ml/` The Association of Cancer Online Resources site lists more than 85 cancer information and support mailing lists. In one week, ACOR delivers 1.5 million individual emails across the globe.

➤ `http://www.betterhealth.com/allhealth/boards/` iVillage's Better Health site offers message boards on various types of cancers and related concerns.

How to Research the Medical Literature

We don't blame you for being intimidated by the medical literature, especially if you've never been trained to find it, read it, or understand it. Fortunately, cancer survivor and CancerGuide Webmaster Steve Dunn has invented the wheel for you in his article, "How to Research the Medical Literature" (`http://cancerguide.org/research.html`). Dunn teaches you how to use databases and online resources. This invaluable article explains different types of databases and resources, differences you'll encounter when using them, and the information you'll find from each.

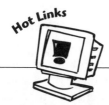

Hot Links

Where to Get Cancer Information Online

`http://www.cancerguide.org/online.html`

Starting your online exploration of cancer resources can be daunting. Your first stop should be this "tour of important Internet sites for getting basic information on your cancer." You'll learn about the three major sites, plus the best mailing lists and newsgroups.

Start Here: General Cancer Info Sites

Even though we told you that you could find 1.5 million cancer sites (and that was just with one search engine), some clear winners emerge as the places to start. All of our Medical Super Sites have good cancer resources. In addition, the following sites specialize in cancer, and are comprehensive and trustworthy.

American Cancer Society

`http://www.cancer.org`

What is cancer? Am I at risk for cancer? How can I tell whether I have cancer? What should I ask my doctor? What happens after treatment? You get all your questions answered at this colossal site. Read about risk factors, prevention, diagnostic techniques, the latest treatment options, alternative and complementary methods, and living with cancer, and visit ACS's bookstore.

CancerNet

`http://wwwicic.nci.nih.gov/patient.htm`

This is the National Cancer Institute's (NCI) Web site for cancer patients and the public. Updated monthly, all information is reviewed by oncology experts and is based on current research. The PDQ section (click **treatment information**, or go directly to `http://wwwicic.nci.nih.gov/clinpdq/pif.html`) lists cancers alphabetically, clearly and simply, describing prevention, detection, treatment, and supportive care for each.

CancerGuide

http://www.cancerguide.org

This site takes you by the hand and teaches you how to research your cancer. Start with "Tour of CancerGuide," which shows you how to find the specific information you want. Then explore the extensive site to learn about cancer and your situation, helpful books, confronting a difficult diagnosis, stories of other patients, clinical trials, treatments, how to research the medical literature, specific cancers, and alternative therapies. This site was created by Steve Dunn, a cancer patient from Boulder, Colorado, who has done scads of work on your behalf.

OncoLink

http://cancer.med.upenn.edu

OncoLink, a well-respected site from the University of Pennsylvania Cancer Center, has a wealth of information: specific types of cancer, medical specialties that deal with cancer, chemotherapy, bone marrow transplants, ways to cope with cancer, shared experiences of patients and survivors, causes, screening, prevention, clinical trials, financial issues, artwork, and additional resources. It's all here.

Ask NOAH About: Cancer

http://www.noah.cuny.edu/cancer/cancer.html

You'll find dozens of categories and hundreds of articles and links on this popular site from New York Online Access to Health (NOAH), providing "high-quality, full-text health information for consumers that is accurate, timely, relevant, and unbiased." NOAH is a team project from the City University of New York, the Metropolitan New York Library Council, the New York Academy of Medicine, and the New York Public Library.

CanSearch: Online Guide to Cancer Resources

http://www.cansearch.org/canserch/canserch.htm

"The purpose of CanSearch is to assist online users in finding Internet cancer resources. CanSearch will take you step by step to each of the storehouses of cancer information. Many of the Internet sites are true gold mines of information." This site, from the National Coalition for Cancer Survivorship, is itself a gold mine, with reviewed resources about basic research, clinical trials, support, dealing with pain, end-of-life issues, general cancer publications, specific types of cancer, other sources of support, and gaining inspiration.

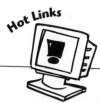

Hot Links

American Cancer Society Web Resources

`http://www2.cancer.org/wwwDir.cfm`

Find links to sites reviewed by the American Cancer Society on a variety of cancers, plus clinical trials, alternative medicine, support, and more.

Specific Cancers

You can't go wrong with the sites listed above. If you're looking for more information about a specific cancer, the following sites are also outstanding resources.

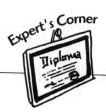

Expert's Corner

"Regular mammograms are important because they identify breast abnormalities that may be cancer long before physical symptoms develop. Numerous studies have shown that early detection saves lives and increases a woman's treatment options."

—Robert Smith, Ph.D., Director, Cancer Screening, American Cancer Society

Breast Cancer

Women fear breast cancer more than any other disease (although heart disease and lung cancer kill more women than breast cancer). An enormous number of resources are now available—online and offline—for information and support, including the following outstanding Web sites.

NCCN Breast Cancer Treatment Guidelines for Patients

http://www.cancernetwork.com/guidelines/Breast/Page1.htm

The National Comprehensive Cancer Network and the American Cancer Society offer specific, state-of-the-art recommendations for treating women with breast cancer written by experts from 17 leading cancer centers.

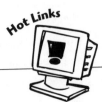

Hot Links

Diary of a Mastectomy: Surviving the Bad News

http://underwire.msn.com/Underwire/bodyworks/be/72eclectic.asp

"Breast cancer catapults its victims onto a mental roller-coaster ride. Neck-jerking curves. Dizzying drops into dark tunnels. Long, slow uphill grinds." Read Sharon Sorenson's riveting personal story about breast cancer.

National Alliance of Breast Cancer Organizations (NABCO)

www.nabco.org

Do breast implants cause disease? Should healthy breasts be removed if there is a family history of breast cancer? This site from NABCO, a network of breast-cancer organizations, offers news, resources, clinical trials, and support.

Breast Health

http://www.breastcancerinfo.com/bhealth/

This warm and welcoming site from the Susan G. Komen Breast Cancer Foundation presents facts about breast health, strategies for living with breast cancer, and much more (see Figure 20.2).

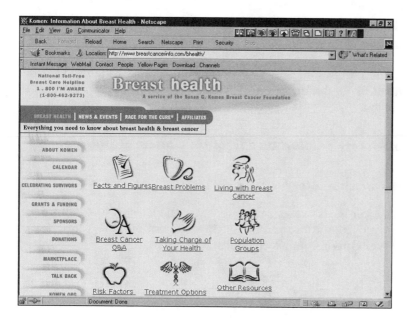

Figure 20.2

The Susan G. Komen Breast Cancer Foundation offers facts and support.

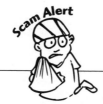

Scam Alert

Breast Cancer and Antiperspirant: The Truth

http://www2.cancer.org/zine/dsp_StoryIndex.cfm?fn=001_05211999_0

Contrary to the email that's circulating, breast cancer is not caused by antiperspirant. Read how the American Cancer Society picks apart this email line by line. The moral of the story: Never believe or circulate an email health scare without checking out the evidence at a reputable site.

Colon Cancer

Colon cancer (also known as colorectal cancer) is the second leading cause of death from cancer in the United States—lung cancer is first. Colon cancer is an equal-opportunity cancer that strikes both men and women. Catching this cancer early is the key to cure and survival. Learn more from the following sites.

Dr. Dan Talks to You About Colorectal Cancer

http://www.gastro.org/drdan-colc.html

"Dr. Dan" answers common questions about colorectal cancer in this site from the American Digestive Health Foundation, complete with illustrations of the digestive system and colonic polyps.

American Cancer Society's Colon and Rectum Cancer Resource Center

http://www3.cancer.org/cancerinfo/res_home.asp?ct=10

Learn what colorectal cancer is, its causes and risk factors, the latest strategies for prevention, new diagnostic techniques, and the latest treatment options. Click **Colorectal Cancer Overview** for an excellent introduction.

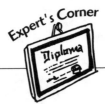

Expert's Corner

"Many colorectal cancers can be prevented, and finding them early is the best way to improve the chance of a cure and reduce the number of deaths caused by this disease."

—Gabriel Feldman, M.D., Director, Prostate and Colorectal Cancer Control, American Cancer Society

Lung Cancer

Lung cancer is the number one killer cancer, and the cancer that is the most easily prevented. Learn about it from the following sites. Also see the "Kicking Butts: Smoking Cessation" section of Chapter 12, "Getting Unhooked: Fighting Addictions," for terrific smoking-cessation Web sites.

Alliance for Lung Cancer Advocacy, Support, and Education (ALCASE)

http://www.alcase.org/

ALCASE's mission is to help people with lung cancer improve their quality of life. Click **Lung Cancer Manual** for a 200-page online book about lung cancer. (Don't worry, you can read one chapter at a time.) Click **Lung Cancer Support** for support groups, phone buddies, and stories of hope.

Waging War on Lung Cancer

http://www.fda.gov/fdac/features/1999/399_lung.html

This detailed article from *FDA Consumer* magazine explains diagnosis, treatment, risks, warning signs, stages, and the future of lung-cancer research.

Lung Cancer

http://cancernet.nci.nih.gov/wyntk_pubs/lung.htm

This online booklet from the National Cancer Institute discusses lung-cancer causes, prevention, symptoms, detection, diagnosis, and treatment.

Ovarian Cancer

Each year ovarian cancer is diagnosed in about 26,000 women in the United States. This is a difficult cancer to detect early. Learn about ovarian cancer from the following sites.

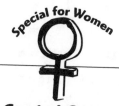

Special for Women

Cervical Cancer

http://www.wcn.org/about/cervical.html

Read a series of articles from the Women's Cancer Network, presented by the Gynecology Cancer Foundation, including facts about cervical cancer, factors that increase or decrease your risk, diagnosis, and treatment.

Ovarian Cancer

http://www.fda.gov/opacom/catalog/ovarian.html

This article from the RDA describes Gilda Radner's struggle with ovarian cancer, the importance of early detection, methods for diagnosis, and treatment options.

Gilda Radner Ovarian Cancer Registry

`http://rpci.med.buffalo.edu/clinic/gynonc/grwp.html`

Learn what ovarian cancer is, and read about risks, family history, and Q&As from the Gilda Radner Familial Ovarian Cancer Registry at Roswell Park Cancer Institute.

National Ovarian Cancer Coalition (NOCC)

`http://www.ovarian.org/main.html`

This site has a variety of ovarian-cancer resources: a fact sheet, articles, resources, personal stories, and plenty of support.

Prostate Cancer

One out of every six men is at lifetime risk for prostate cancer, according to CaP CURE, which funds prostate-cancer research. All men (and the women who love them) need to educate themselves about this cancer, and the following sites can help.

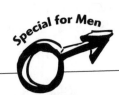

Special for Men

How to Do a Testicular Self Examination

`http://www.acor.org/diseases/TC/tcexam.html`

Monthly self-exams of the testicles help you detect testicular cancer at an early stage when it is very curable. This illustrated guide from the National Cancer Institute shows you exactly how to do it.

CapCure: About Prostate Cancer

`http://205.139.28.245/aboutprostate/index.html`

"The more you know about prostate cancer, the better equipped you are to fight it." This site has abundant, well-illustrated information—a good starting place.

Prostate Cancer: No One Answer for Testing or Treatment

http://www.fda.gov/fdac/features/1998/598_pros.html

Learn the facts about diagnosing and treating prostate cancer and benign prostatic hyperplasia in this helpful, simply written guide from the FDA.

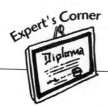

Expert's Corner

"Getting information about prostate cancer is one thing about this disease that can be easy. Physicians, families, and friends can be a valuable support network by helping men obtain accurate, current information. The power of this knowledge is the best weapon in overcoming prostate cancer fear and confusion—and that makes us all better at fighting this disease."

—Gabriel Feldman, M.D., Director, Prostate and Colorectal Cancer Control, American Cancer Society

Prostate Cancer InfoLink

http://www.comed.com/Prostate/

This site has everything: a ton of clearly written information about all aspects of prostate cancer, plus Q&As, support organizations, and mailing lists.

What to Do If Prostate Cancer Strikes: A Helpbook

http://www.cancerresearch.org/prostatebook.html

This site from the American Cancer Society and the Cancer Research Institute explains why there is hope, how to choose a therapy, experimental treatments, and offers additional resources.

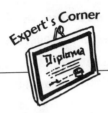

Skin Cancer

Our love affair with the sun has put many of us at risk for skin cancer. Learn how to avoid, recognize, and treat skin cancer from the following sites.

Skin Cancer Foundation

`http://www.skincancer.org/`

Everything you want to know about skin cancer is here, including helpful photographs of the warning signs of melanoma, basal cell carcinoma, and squamous cell carcinoma.

American Academy of Dermatology

`http://www.aad.org/`

Click **Patient Information** to see a list of articles on skin cancer and how to protect yourself from it from the American Academy of Dermatology.

Thwarting Skin Cancer with Sun Sense

`http://www.fda.gov/fdac/features/695_skincanc.html`

This article from the FDA explains how to protect yourself from skin cancer with strategies for avoiding sun exposure and tanning devices.

Seven Steps to Safer Sunning

`http://www.fda.gov/fdac/features/596_7sun.html`

This *FDA Consumer* reprint describes seven "safer sun practices" recommended by the American Academy of Dermatology, American Cancer Society, Skin Cancer Foundation, and other medical experts.

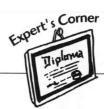

Expert's Corner

Diploma

"Be aware of sun exposure and skin cancer. Remember that your skin has memory, so that bad sunburns that occurred in the past still have the damaged and abnormal cells that may turn cancerous with much more sun exposure. Sun ages the skin more than anything. For these reasons, use a good sunscreen that blocks UVA and UVB, at least a number SPF 15. Put on at least 2 to 4 tablespoons and massage it in thoroughly to all the sun exposed areas. Apply this every 3 to 4 hours or when in and out of the water. This is true for casual sun exposure (which means gardening, walking, sports). Try to forget about sun tanning altogether."

—James J. Romano, M.D., cosmetic surgeon (`http://www.jromano.com`)

The Least You Need to Know

➤ You can find trustworthy information online about every kind of cancer.

➤ Start with the most reputable medical and cancer organizations.

➤ Be wary of treatments with unproven benefits.

➤ Take advantage of the many cancer support groups available online.

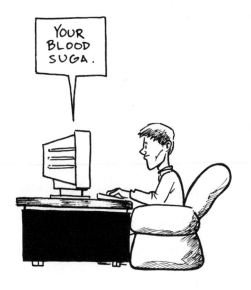

Diabetes

Billie Jean King, Jackie Robinson, Catfish Hunter, and Arthur Ashe didn't let diabetes stop them from excelling in sports. Diabetes didn't slow down the show biz careers of Jack Benny, Mae West, or James Cagney, or stop the music of Ella Fitzgerald, Elvis Presley, or Giacomo Puccini. It didn't prevent Thomas Edison from inventing, Paul Cézanne from painting, or Ernest Hemingway from writing.

The point is that you can live a productive, high-quality life with diabetes. This is especially true with today's medical advances.

The Internet provides all sorts of resources for learning about diabetes, managing it, talking to other people with diabetes, and helping children cope with their conditions. This chapter introduces you to some of the best sites for information, advice, and support.

Learning About Diabetes

Diabetes is a disease characterized by the inability of the body to produce or to respond to insulin to maintain proper blood glucose levels. That means that the body either doesn't make enough insulin—the hormone that helps glucose (blood sugar) get into the cells—or can't use its own insulin efficiently, so sugars build up in the blood.

Warning Signs

If you think you or a family member might have diabetes, an appointment with a physician is essential for diagnosis. Warning signs might include some of the following symptoms, but a person can have diabetes without any of these warning signs:

➤ Frequent urination

➤ Extreme thirst

➤ Unexplained weight loss

➤ Extreme hunger

➤ Sudden vision changes

➤ Tingling or numbness in hands or feet

➤ Feeling exhausted much of the time

➤ Excessively dry skin

➤ Slow-healing sores

➤ Frequent infections

Types

The major types of diabetes are the following:

➤ **Type 1 diabetes (previously called insulin-dependent diabetes mellitus or juvenile-onset diabetes)**   The body stops producing insulin, requiring insulin injections. Type 1 diabetes might account for 5 to 10 percent of diagnosed cases of diabetes.

➤ **Type 2 diabetes (previously called non-insulin-dependent diabetes mellitus or adult-onset diabetes)**   The body still produces insulin but does not use it properly. Type 2 diabetes might account for about 90 to 95 percent of all diagnosed cases of diabetes.

After you have been diagnosed and know what type you have, learn more from the American Diabetes Association (`http://diabetes.org/ada/c20a.asp` for Type 1 or `http://diabetes.org/ada/c20b.asp` for Type 2).

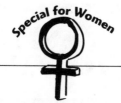

Diabetes: Take It Seriously

http://www.obgyn.net/english/pubs/features/tfp/diabetes.htm

This clear guide by Geneva Collins, originally published in *The Female Patient*, helps women understand Type 2 diabetes: the importance of early diagnosis, treatment, and its impact on pregnancy and menopause.

Start Here: First-Step Sites for Learning About Diabetes

If you or a loved one has just been diagnosed, let the following sites be your learning centers.

Frequently Asked Questions

http://www.cdc.gov/nccdphp/ddt/faqs.htm

This site from the Centers for Disease Control is a good starting place to get an overview of what diabetes is, its symptoms, types, risk factors, treatment, prevention, and resources.

American Diabetes Association

http://diabetes.org/

The American Diabetes Association's mission is "to prevent and cure diabetes, and to improve the lives of all people affected by diabetes." Bookmark this page for news, treatment information, recipes, exercise tips, and dozens of articles to help you understand diabetes and live a rich, healthy life. If you've just been diagnosed, click **Newly Diagnosed** as your first stop.

Beginner's Guide to Diabetes

http://www.joslin.harvard.edu/education/beginnerguide.html

This site from the Joslin Diabetes Center offers a variety of articles to help you educate yourself when you or a loved one has been diagnosed with diabetes (see Figure 21.1).

Figure 21.1

*If you've just been diag-
nosed, visit the Joslin
Diabetes Center Web site.*

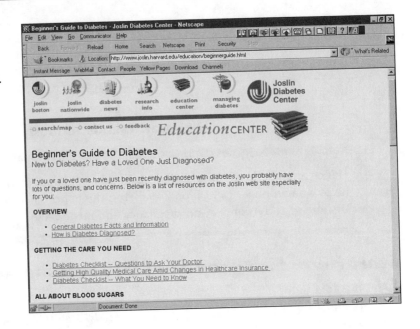

Living with Diabetes

After you have educated yourself about the basics, you'll want to delve deeper into
ways to manage your diabetes and live a productive, quality life. Whether you're
looking for medical supplies or exploring a targeted topic, you'll find information at
the following special sites.

Ask NOAH About: Diabetes

http://www.noah.cuny.edu/diabetes/diabetes.html

New York Online Access to Health (NOAH) presents screened links to keep you clicking and reading for months. The links are categorized so you easily find the exact
topic you seek, whether it's diabetes and pregnancy, alternative treatments, or foot
care.

Useful Addresses

http://www.drrubin.com/addresses.html

Alan L. Rubin, M.D., offers reviewed links to every type of diabetes Web site imaginable. You find all the major sites, plus sites for buying diabetes products, sites for the
visually impaired, and even sites about diabetic pets. It's a gold mine.

Treatment

Medicine has come a long way in treating diabetes. Explore the information you find at reputable sites on the Web, then take that information to discuss with your doctor.

OnHealth Diabetes Center

http://onhealth.com/ch1/condctr/diabetes/item%2c28.asp

"The wealth of ideas and information in this condition center can help you meet the challenges of diabetes and live a healthier life." This patient guide from OnHealth in association with the International Diabetes Center covers tests, treatments, meters, health tips, and recipes.

Diabetes & Other Endocrine Conditions

http://www.mayohealth.org/mayo/library/htm/tocdiabe.htm

This site from the Mayo Clinic library offers drug updates, diabetes management, complications prevention, and more.

Blood Glucose Monitoring: Your Tool for Diabetes Control

http://www.joslin.harvard.edu/education/library/monitor.htm

Learn why, when, and how to check your blood glucose in this informative guide from the Joslin Diabetes Center.

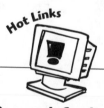

Hot Links

Research Studies

http://www.niddk.nih.gov/

If you're interested in getting involved in a diabetes study, click **Patient Recruitment** to learn which research studies need patients. The site is run by the National Institute of Diabetes and Digestive and Kidney Diseases (NIDDK), part of the National Institutes of Health (NIH).

Lifestyle

Eating right and exercise are both parts of a healthy lifestyle for people with diabetes. The following sites help you know what you're doing.

Diabetes.com

http://www.diabetes.com/

This site "empowers diabetics to manage the disease more confidently, effectively, and economically," published by PlanetRx. It provides plenty of information, plus support groups. (see Figure 21.2).

Figure 21.2

Diabetes.com provides a wealth of information and support.

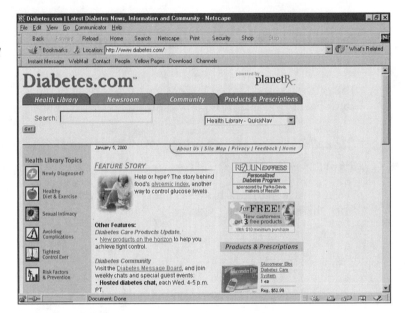

20 Steps to Safe Exercise

http://diabetes.org/ada/c40j.asp

"Exercise helps pep up insulin's action." These 20 steps from the American Diabetes Association help you exercise safely, pleasurably, and effectively.

There's No Such Thing as a "Diabetic Diet"

http://www.joslin.harvard.edu/education/library/nodiet2.html

There's a lot of outdated information and misinformation about what people with diabetes should and shouldn't eat. Smash the myths with this article from the Joslin Diabetes Center.

I Have Diabetes: What Should I Eat?

http://www.niddk.nih.gov/health/diabetes/pubs/nutritn/what/index.htm

This comprehensive, yet simple, nutritional guide is from the National Diabetes Information Clearinghouse. The illustrations and forms that you fill out help to clarify and personalize the information even more.

Nutrition

http://diabetes.org/nutrition/

The nutrition section of the American Diabetes Association Web site offers a nutrition guide, recipes, cookbook recommendations, articles, and healthy restaurant eating.

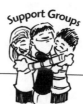

Online Diabetes Resources

http://www.mendosa.com/faq.htm

"Tracking Diabetes on the Web Since February 1995," journalist Rick Mendosa compiles and reviews 56 international diabetes mailing lists (with specifics about how to subscribe), 20 message boards, and a variety of newsgroups and chats.

The Complications

http://onhealth.com/ch1/condctr/diabetes/item,132.asp

Read about diabetes complications and damage, and how to prevent them. This detailed patient guide is from OnHealth's Diabetes Center in association with the International Diabetes Center.

Avoiding Complications

http://www.diabetes.com/health_library/avoiding_complications.html

This section of Diabetes.com explains the major complications of diabetes and how to avoid and control them.

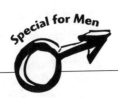

Men's Sexual Health

`http://www.diabetes.org/ada/c50b.asp`

Impotence occurs among 50 to 60 percent of men with diabetes over the age of 50. This article from the American Diabetes Association explains the connection between diabetes and impotence and what you can do about it.

Children with Diabetes

Your first reaction to finding out that your child has diabetes might be panic and distress. Ease your mind by educating yourself. Learn the facts about childhood diabetes and how you can help your child cope with this condition. The following sites can help.

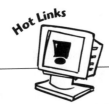

Babysitting Guidelines

`http://www.childrenwithdiabetes.com/d_02_900.htm`

Print out this excellent guide for babysitting a child with diabetes, and give it to your babysitter.

Children with Diabetes

`http://www.childrenwithdiabetes.com/`

"The on-line community for kids, families, and adults with diabetes" has plenty of information and support for children with diabetes and their parents. Originally created by the father of a diabetic child, the site has grown into a huge repository of information overseen by medical advisors.

Kids Learn About Diabetes

`http://www.geocities.com/HotSprings/6935/index.html`

Written by kids for kids (all information cleared by an endocrinologist), this site uses simple language to give a tutorial on diabetes, including complications, shots, healthy diet, and fears and feelings. This site started as an Eagle Scout service project by Brendan Hannemann of Troop 1140, Springfield, Virginia.

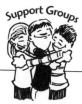

People

`http://www.childrenwithdiabetes.com/people/`

Children with Diabetes offers lots of support: kids telling their stories, pen pals, art, message board, chat rooms, and mailing lists.

The Least You Need to Know

➤ You can find clear, reputable information about diabetes online.

➤ The Web can help you explore treatments and keep a healthy lifestyle.

➤ Children with diabetes can learn about their condition and find support online.

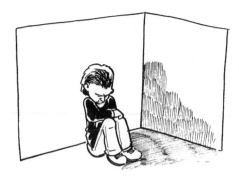

Chapter 22

Depression

In This Chapter

➤ Recognizing symptoms of depression

➤ Understanding depression as an illness

➤ Exploring treatment options online

What do Abraham Lincoln, Theodore Roosevelt, Robert Schumann, Ludwig von Beethoven, Edgar Allen Poe, Mark Twain, Vincent van Gogh, and Georgia O'Keefe all have in common? They all suffered from depression.

Depression hits about 17 million American adults every year, according to the National Institute of Mental Health (NIMH). That's more than heart disease, cancer, or AIDS.

If you or a loved one lives with depression, this chapter is a valuable aid for finding online resources for learning about this condition, getting professional help, and finding compassionate support.

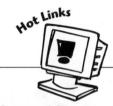

General Depression

`http://www.nimh.nih.gov/depression/genpop.htm`

The National Institute of Mental Health explains depression—symptoms, diagnosis, treatment, and where to get help.

Diagnosis

We all have times of feeling down in the dumps. How often have you proclaimed, "I'm depressed!" when you felt blue? As awful as the emotional dark hours seem at the moment, it might just take a good cry, a night's sleep, a trashy novel, or a pint of Rocky Road ice cream to set things right.

Other times, you might sink into gloom for a period of time—when a relationship ends, a loved one dies, or you lose your job. Generally, time heals these wounds, or at least makes them recede enough that you can function normally and move on with your life.

People who are truly depressed, however, don't bounce back. Their illness can be incapacitating, fierce, distressing, and sometimes life threatening. Depression is a serious illness that doesn't go away by itself and needs to be diagnosed and treated by a medical professional.

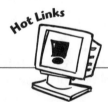

Dealing with the Depths of Depression

`http://www.fda.gov/fdac/features/1998/498_dep.html`

Start your exploration by reading this article from the U.S. Food and Drug Administration. It is a clear and positive overview of what depression is, how it feels, who gets it and why, and how it is treated.

Symptoms

If you or a loved one has these symptoms of depression from the American Psychiatric Association's *Diagnostic and Statistical Manual*, please seek professional help:

➤ Depressed mood

➤ Loss of interest or pleasure in almost all activities

➤ Changes in appetite or weight

➤ Disturbed sleep

➤ Slowed or restless movements

➤ Fatigue, loss of energy

➤ Feelings of worthlessness or excessive guilt

➤ Trouble in thinking, concentrating, or making decisions

➤ Recurrent thoughts of death or suicide

Are You Depressed?

If the symptoms you just read make you worry that you or someone you know might be depressed, you can learn more clues online. Realize that questionnaires, self-tests, and symptom lists are just indicators that there's enough of a problem to see a professional. They do not substitute for professional diagnosis. (Have I repeated this enough, yet?)

Depression Questionnaire

http://mentalhelp.net/guide/dep2quiz.htm

This 18-question questionnaire, known as the Goldberg Depression Inventory, can help you determine if you need to see a mental health professional for diagnosis and treatment of depression. You might want to take this test weekly to track your moods, and then share this information with your health professional.

Depression Can Lurk Beneath the Surface

http://www.healthcentral.com/drdean/DeanFullTextTopics.cfm?ID=17967

Do you know an older person who might be depressed, even though he or she doesn't necessarily act sad? Dr. Dean Edell describes clinical clues that reveal underlying depression in older adults.

Let's Talk About Depression

http://www.nimh.nih.gov/depression/genpop/letstalk.htm

This article from the National Institute of Mental Health helps teenagers look at whether they or a friend might be depressed, with advice and strategies for doing something about it.

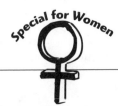

Special for Women

Mental Health Learning Center for Women

http://www.womens-health.com/health_center/mental/index.html

Women are twice as likely as men to become depressed, according to the National Institute of Mental Health (NIMH). Assess your knowledge of this illness. Then read a variety of articles about depression with a focus on women, such as female biology and depression, and the types of depression that affect women particularly.

Suicide Prevention

Approximately 30 percent of clinically depressed people attempt suicide, and about half of them succeed in killing themselves. If you or a loved one is contemplating suicide, please seek professional help. The following resources do not substitute for a live professional, but they provide additional help when you need it at any hour, and in complete privacy.

Suicide: Read This First

http://www.metanoia.org/suicide/

This warm, earnest, and well-crafted letter is a deterrent to suicide because it acknowledges the pain and shares strategies for getting through the crisis. This site has links to additional online resources. If you are helping a person who is suicidal, go to http://www.metanoia.org/suicide/whattodo.htm.

The Samaritans

http://www.samaritans.org.uk/

The Samaritans is a non-religious charity founded in 1953 that exists "to provide confidential emotional support to any person who is suicidal or despairing." Trained volunteers read and reply to emails daily.

Types

There are several types of depression, and you can find plenty of information about each one on the World Wide Web. The following are the main types:

➤ **Major Depression**   Major depression is an episode or ongoing condition of disabling gloom that interferes with the ability to work, sleep, eat, and enjoy activities that used to be pleasurable. Learn more from *Finding Peace of Mind: Medication Strategies for Depression*, an online booklet from the National Depressive and Manic-Depressive Association at http://www.ndmda.org/peacedep.htm.

➤ **Dysthymia**   A Greek word meaning "bad state of mind," dysthymia is a less intense form of depression, but it might last longer and become more severe.

➤ **Bipolar Depression**   Also known as manic-depression, bipolar depression is characterized by "extreme mood swings from overly 'high' and irritable (mania) to sad and hopeless (depression) and then back again, with periods of normal mood in between," explains Mental Health Net at http://bipolar.mentalhelp.net/. This site also offers *Your Complete Well-Connected Guide to Bipolar Disorder* at http://bipolar.mentalhelp.net/bipolar/wcg_bipolar_toc.htm.

Treatment

Eighty to 90 percent of cases of depression can be treated effectively, according to the American Psychiatric Association (APA). Unfortunately, two-thirds of the people suffering from depression don't get the help they need. Many don't recognize the severity of their symptoms, or chalk them up to lack of sleep or a poor diet. Fatigue and shame stop others from seeking help.

Psychotherapy and medications are effective treatments for depression, especially in combination. They can shorten the length of time you feel depressed, and prevent recurrences. Researching treatments on the Web is one potent way of taking back control and feeling more in charge.

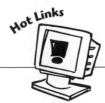

Treatment: Major Depressive Disorder

http://mentalhelp.net/disorders/sx22t.htm

Learn about different types of psychotherapy and medications that are effective for the treatment of major depression from Mental Health Net. The style here is a bit stiff, but the information is worthwhile.

Talk Therapy

Psychotherapy is talking guided by a qualified therapist. Although you can find online therapists who "talk" to you via email, that's best for less severe emotional problems, not clinical depression. A reputable online therapist will recommend that you see a one-on-one, live therapist if your depression goes deeper than a temporary emotional setback. If you get that advice, don't fight it—take it.

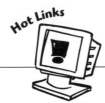

Mood Disorders: Depression & Manic Depression

http://www.nami.org/disorder/disord6.htm

This online pamphlet from the National Alliance for the Mentally Ill discusses depression and manic depression, how they might affect your life, and how they can be treated, with plenty of clear information about medications.

Antidepressant Medications

A variety of medications, called antidepressants, are effective for treating depression, and your personal psychiatrist or physician is the best person to advise you. Though you must not self-medicate from the Internet (please!), you can inform yourself about the effects of different antidepressant medications and discuss your findings with your health professional. People who are depressed often feel powerless and out of control.

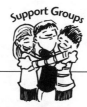

Depression Support Groups

One of the worst parts of depression is the feeling of isolation. An online support group can make you feel connected and give you a community that understands what you're going through.

➤ `http://www.support-group.com/` Click **depression** to see a list of depression support groups: bulletin boards, Usenet groups, mailing lists, and supportive articles. This site also has information about "live" support groups in your local area, and articles providing support.

➤ `http://mentalhelp.net/bipolar/online.htm` Mental Health Net offers forums and chats for people with bipolar disorder.

➤ `http://drkoop.com/conditions/Depression/` Dr. Koop's site offers chats and message boards, with a clearly stated, strict privacy policy.

➤ `http://mentalhelp.net/depression/online.htm` Mental Health Net provides links to additional online support resources.

Start Here: Depression Info Sites

Depression

`http://depression.mentalhelp.net/`

You are not alone, and you are not to blame. "Depression is not a character flaw, nor is it simply feeling blue for a few days. Most importantly, depression is not your fault." Mental Health Net helps you understand this condition, its causes, and its treatments (see Figure 22.1). The annotated links will keep you reading for days.

Figure 22.1

Mental Health Net offers a wealth of information about depression.

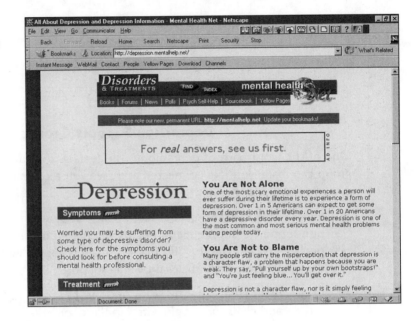

National Depressive and Manic-Depressive Association

www.ndmda.org

The National Depressive and Manic-Depressive Association is a patient-run organization providing support and education to people with depression. Use this site to find information and a local, live chapter to keep current on the latest in treatment methods, find recommended mental health professionals in your area, and share your feelings in a confidential and supportive setting.

National Alliance for the Mentally Ill

www.nami.org

The National Alliance for the Mentally Ill is a grassroots, self-help support and advocacy organization. NAMI's mission is "to eradicate mental illness and to improve the quality of life for those who suffer from these no-fault brain diseases." Type **depression** in the search box and you get hundreds of clearly written, supportive, and informative articles from NAMI.

National Institute of Mental Health

www.nimh.nih.gov

This site from the National Institute of Mental Health (NIMH) has notices about clinical trials, reviews of new antidepressants, and online brochures about depression.

Andrew's Depression Page

`http://www.blarg.net/~charlatn/Depression.html`

Andrew Fineberg chronicles his personal battle with depression (click **How I Am** for his Depression Treatment Timeline with occasional updates since 1994), information about depression, and many links to other helpful sites.

HealthFinder.com

`http://www.healthfinder.com`

Are you looking for something more specific than general information about depression? Type **depression** in the search box, and you get a list of reviewed Web resources and organizations on related subjects, including depression and the elderly, postpartum depression, and the depressed child.

The Least You Need to Know

➤ Depression is a serious illness; it's not the same as feeling blue or temporarily down.

➤ You can learn about the types of depression, symptoms, and treatments online.

➤ Although you can learn about depression on the Internet, professional help is essential to overcoming it.

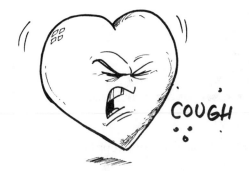

Chapter 23

Heart Disease

In This Chapter

➤ Exploring how your heart works, and how to keep it healthy

➤ Heart-disease risks and how to prevent them

➤ Learning about heart attacks online

Coronary heart disease is America's number one killer for both men and women. The World Wide Web is an extraordinary source of information, whether you have a healthy heart and want to keep it that way, or you're managing risks, or you've had a heart attack and want to understand all you can about preventing another one.

This chapter gives you an introduction to heart health and shows you where to find information on an array of heart topics.

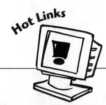

Anatomy and Physiology of the Cardiovascular System

http://www.merck.com/disease/heart/anatomy/

What does a heart look like, and how does it work? Learn about your heart, blood vessels, and blood with this illustrated guide.

Prevention

Your heart is an extraordinary organ that pumps blood continuously. Although the heart is no bigger than a fist, it is powerful enough to send oxygen and nourishment to all the muscles and organs of the body.

When the heart is healthy, it adjusts to different demands, providing more or less blood as needed. During rest, it pumps from 5 to 6 quarts of blood a minute; during exercise, it beats faster and can pump more than 20 quarts a minute.

If you have heart disease, your heart is weaker and can't pump as much blood with each beat as a healthy heart.

You can't change all your risk factors for heart disease, such as older age or a family history of heart disease. However, the following are risk factors that you *can* change or control:

➤ Smoking

➤ High blood pressure

➤ High blood cholesterol

➤ Inactive lifestyle

➤ Overweight

➤ Diabetes

➤ Stress

Although your genes play a huge role in your risk of developing heart disease, there's plenty you can do to lower your risk, such as quitting smoking, lowering your cholesterol, eating healthy, and exercising.

For heart-healthy eating, exercising, and weight loss, *The Complete Idiot's Guide to Online Health and Fitness* by Joan Price and Shannon Entin is a terrific resource. The following sites can also help you make some lifestyle changes for your heart's sake.

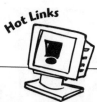

Hot Links

Preventing Heart Disease: Making Lifestyle Changes

http://www.ama-assn.org/insight/yourhlth/heartrsk/changes.htm

Making lifestyle changes can be difficult. This guide from the American Medical Association helps you look at your readiness to make a change and some first steps for making your heart healthier.

Quitting Smoking

Smoking causes almost as many deaths from heart disease as from lung cancer. Women who smoke, for example, are two to six times more likely to suffer a heart attack than nonsmoking women, and the risk increases with the number of cigarettes you smoke each day, according to the National Heart, Lung, and Blood Institute. Smoking also boosts the risk of stroke.

To help you quit, see the "Kicking Butts: Smoking Cessation" section of Chapter 12, "Getting Unhooked: Fighting Addictions." For the specific link between smoking and heart disease, see the following site.

Facts About Heart Disease and Women: Kicking the Smoking Habit

http://www.nhlbi.nih.gov/health/public/heart/other/hdw_smk.htm

This guide explains why your heart needs you to quit smoking, and gives practical tips for breaking the habit. This National Heart, Lung, and Blood Institute fact sheet is available in PDF or ASCII format.

Exercise

Physical activity is a powerful heart strengthener. *The Complete Idiot's Guide to Online Health and Fitness* by Joan Price and Shannon Entin tells you how to find the best online exercise information. Meanwhile, the following sites can get you started.

FitnessLink

http://www.fitnesslink.com

Your heart needs exercise to get and stay strong. FitnessLink is your exercise resource, with articles, advice, guidelines, motivation, and support to get you moving and enjoying it (see Figure 23.1).

Figure 23.1

Whatever you want to know about exercise and fitness, you can learn from FitnessLink.

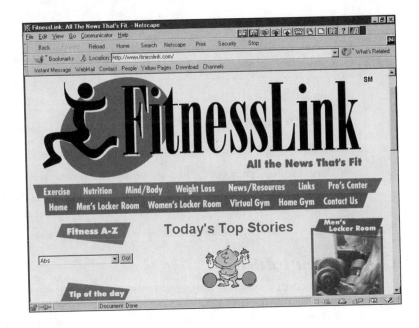

Joan Price's Web Site

`http://www.joanprice.com`

Okay, I'm tooting my own horn, but helping people get lively is my business, so please visit my site and read the many articles I've written to help you make exercise a habit. Your heart will thank you.

More Prevention Help

The following sites give you more strategies for preventing heart disease.

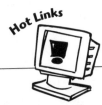

Hot Links

An Aspirin a Day...Just a Cliché?

`http://www.fda.gov/fdac/features/1999/299_asp.html`

Should you take an aspirin to avoid a heart attack or stroke? This article from the FDA explains when, why, and how much.

Live Healthier, Live Longer

http://rover.nhlbi.nih.gov/chd/

This site from the National Heart, Lung, and Blood Institute explains the connection between cholesterol and heart disease, and teaches you how to lower your cholesterol.

Preventing Heart Disease Quiz

http://www.ama-assn.org/insight/yourhlth/heartrsk/quiz.htm

This quiz from the American Heart Association helps you identify risks that might increase your chances of developing heart disease.

Diet and Nutrition

http://www.americanheart.org/catalog/Health_catpage4.html

Better food habits can help you reduce your risk for heart attack. The AHA helps you eat right with nutrition facts, dietary guidelines, and recipes.

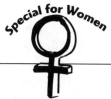

Heart Disease: Biggest Killer of Women

"Heart attacks kill about 235,000 women each year, more than five times the number killed by breast cancer. Breast cancer remains a real problem, but studies consistently show that women overestimate their risk of breast cancer, while drastically underestimating the risk of heart disease. Yet heart disease has been the biggest killer of American women—not from some recent time, but going all the way back to 1908!"

—Charlotte Libov, author of *Beat Your Risk Factors: A Woman's Guide to Reducing Her Risk for Cancer, Heart Disease, Stroke, Diabetes, and Osteoporosis* (Plume, 1999)

Women and Heart Disease

Each year, 370,000 women die of coronary heart disease, making it the number one killer of American women. About 9 million American women suffer from heart disease and a half million women suffer heart attacks each year, according to the National Heart, Lung, and Blood Institute of the National Institutes of Health.

Women have a greater risk of developing heart disease after menopause, when their bodies are producing less estrogen, which seems to offer protection. Women who go through menopause early, either naturally or from surgical removal of the ovaries, have twice the risk of developing heart disease as women of the same age who have not begun menopause.

Most women do not realize that heart disease is their number one risk, probably because most of the research and media attention on heart disease was focused on men until recently. But heart disease is an equal-opportunity killer.

The following sites present heart-disease information aimed at women.

Healthy Heart Handbook for Women

http://www.pueblo.gsa.gov/cic_text/health/healthy-heart/index.html

This clear and comprehensive handbook from the National Heart, Lung, and Blood Institute covers everything you might want to know about heart disease and women: statistics, risk factors, prevention, and steps for survival during an attack.

Facts About Heart Disease and Women: So You Have Heart Disease

http://www.nhlbi.nih.gov/health/public/heart/other/hdw_syh.htm

Get pages of information about heart disease as it affects women from the National Heart, Lung, and Blood Institute. Choose either ASCII (for an unformatted text version) or PDF (for a nicely formatted version).

Heart Disease Management

http://www.womens-health.com/health_center/heart/

This site from Women's Health Interactive includes a cardiac health assessment test, risk factors, nutritional information, and a discussion group—all targeted at women.

Start Here: Heart Disease Info Sites

The following sites are among the best for educating yourself about heart disease with accurate information in simple language.

American Heart Association

http://www.americanheart.org/

The American Heart Association is "dedicated to providing you with education and information on fighting heart disease and stroke." This site has a ton of information about your heart, heart disease, stroke, and staying healthy (see Figure 23.2).

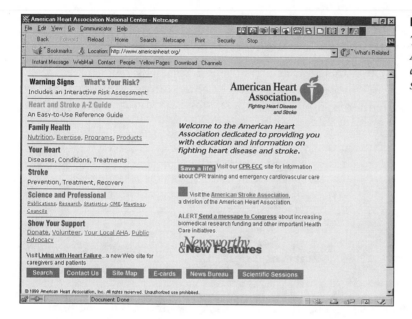

Figure 23.2

The American Heart Association teaches you about heart disease and stroke.

HeartPoint

http://www.heartpoint.com/

"We're here so that you understand your heart, and how to take care of it with the best graphic and written explanations we can muster." This peppy, snazzy site fulfills its promise with information from physicians, physician's assistants, and nurses. Click **HeartPoint Gallery** for animated explanations of a variety of heart topics. This site will keep you interested for hours.

Cardiovascular Information for Patients and the General Public

http://www.nhlbi.nih.gov/health/public/heart/index.htm

This collection of articles from the National Heart, Lung, and Blood Institute includes preventing and controlling high blood pressure, reducing blood cholesterol, and facts about heart disease and women.

Mayo Clinic Heart Center

http://www.mayohealth.org/mayo/common/htm/heartpg.htm

This comprehensive site from the Mayo Clinic includes dozens of articles on reducing risks, treatment, and issues, plus research news, quizzes, links, and heart questions answered by Mayo physicians.

OnHealth Cardiovascular Center

http://onhealth.com/ch1/condctr/cardio/item,14121.asp

This site from OnHealth, in association with the Zena & Michael Wiener Cardiovascular Institute of the Mount Sinai Medical Center, provides information about heart-disease prevention, symptoms, diagnostic tests, conditions, and treatments.

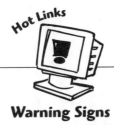

Hot Links

Warning Signs

http://www.americanheart.org/warning.html

What are the warning signs of a heart attack? A stroke? Print out this page from the American Heart Association and make your family memorize it.

Heart Attack

Every 20 seconds, someone in the United States has a heart attack, the most visible and dramatic sign of heart disease. A heart attack—the medical term is myocardial infarction—occurs when the blood supply to the heart muscle stops or is critically decreased. This happens when one of the coronary arteries—the arteries that supply blood to the heart—is blocked.

The following are the most common signs of a heart attack, according to the American Heart Association (http://www.americanheart.org/Heart_and_Stroke_A_Z_Guide/hasy.html):

➤ Uncomfortable pressure, fullness, squeezing, or pain in the center of the chest that lasts more than a few minutes, or goes away and comes back

➤ Pain that spreads to the shoulders, neck or arms

➤ Chest discomfort with lightheadedness, fainting, sweating, nausea or shortness of breath

Less common warning signs of heart attack include other kinds of chest pain, stomach or abdominal pain, nausea, dizziness, shortness of breath, difficulty breathing, anxiety, weakness, fatigue, palpitations, cold sweat, or paleness.

If you're with someone who might be having a heart attack, dial your emergency services number (usually 911) immediately. Expect the person to protest, but quick action is essential.

The following sites teach you about heart attacks: what they are, how to recognize them, and how to respond in an emergency—possibly saving a life.

CPR: You Can Do It!

http://www.heartinfo.com/cpr/cpr.html

If someone has a heart attack, quick action is essential. Take a CPR course to learn what to do, and print out this illustrated guide to memorize and use for reference.

Heart Attack

http://www.americanheart.org/catalog/Heart_catpage19.html

This patient guide from the American Heart Association explains what a heart attack is, prevention guidelines, and diagnostic procedures.

Heart Information Network

http://www.heartinfo.com

This site, founded by a heart patient and a physician, has news and articles about how to prevent, recognize, and treat heart disease (see Figure 23.3). Be sure to click **Heart Attack Warning Signs** and **Heart Attack Guide** for a wealth of information.

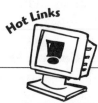

Hot Links

Brain Basics: Preventing Stroke

http://www.ninds.nih.gov/patients/Disorder/STROKE/strokepr.htm

A stroke is a "brain attack" that occurs when blood circulation to the brain fails. Learn about prevention, risk factors, and warning signs from this site from the National Institute of Neurological Disorders and Stroke.

Figure 23.3

Heart Information Network teaches you all about heart disease and prevention.

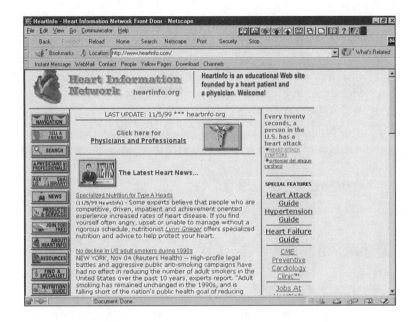

Treatment

Of course your treatment is devised by your doctor, not by a Web site. However, the more you know, the more productive your discussions with your cardiologist can be. The following sites educate you about current treatments. Make a list of questions you want to ask your doctor as you read their content.

Cardiac Treatment

http://www.cardio.com/categories/cardiacarticles.htm#top

Read articles about heart medications and surgeries written by physicians from the Cardiovascular Institute of the South.

OnHealth Cardiovascular Center: Treatments

http://onhealth.com/ch1/condctr/cardio/item,14224.asp

Learn about specific heart surgeries, devices, and medications from this site from OnHealth, in association with the Zena & Michael Wiener Cardiovascular Institute of the Mount Sinai Medical Center.

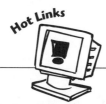

Hot Links

Cardiac Rehabilitation (Consumer's Guide)

http://text.nlm.nih.gov/ftrs/tocview

"Cardiac rehab includes exercise, education, counseling, and learning ways to live a healthier life." This patient guide from the Agency for Health Care Policy and Research (AHCPR) helps people who have had a heart attack or heart surgery recover faster and return to full and productive lives.

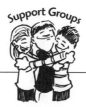

Support Groups

Mended Hearts Support Groups

http://www.mendedhearts.org/purpose.html

Mended Hearts is an extended support group for heart patients, families, and caregivers. Volunteers are people with heart disease who understand what you're going through. They can help you work through the emotions and practical challenges of getting your life back—and then later you can join them in helping others. Mended Hearts is associated with the American Heart Association.

The Least You Need to Know

➤ You can decrease your risk of heart disease through healthy lifestyle choices.

➤ Recognizing the warning signs of heart disease can save your life—or someone else's.

➤ Reputable Web sites can educate you about how to recover from heart attacks and lower your risk of another one.

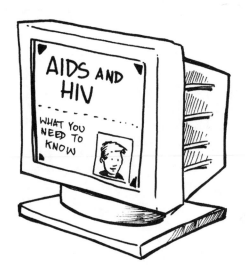

Chapter 24

HIV/AIDS

In This Chapter

➤ Learning about HIV prevention and testing

➤ Online resources for treatments and clinical trials

➤ Cautions to avoid quack cures

Maybe you don't live in one of the large cities with easy access to information about HIV/AIDS where prevention advice and telephone hotline numbers are displayed on bus-stop posters and there are brochures in every library and clinic. Maybe, instead, you live in an isolated area with no easy way to get your questions answered. Or maybe you have reasons for not being able or willing to ask them. Luckily, the Internet obliterates all barriers to gathering accurate and up-to-date information about HIV/AIDS, and this chapter helps you get started.

Prevention

Prevention is the key to stopping the spread of AIDS and keeping yourself safe. You can find safer-sex guidelines, get your questions answered, and learn everything you need to "be prepared."

Prevention Tools

http://www.cdc.gov/nchstp/hiv_aids/prevtools.htm

These articles and reports from the Centers for Disease Control let you delve as deeply into prevention issues as you want. You can find the basics, read about the effectiveness of condoms, and explore a variety of related topics.

Avert

http://www.avert.org

Avert is a British educational and research charity with a mission to "prevent people from becoming infected with HIV, to improve the quality of life for those already infected, and to work with others to develop a cure." This site has a large section aimed at young people. See what you know about AIDS by taking a quiz at http://www.avert.org/hivquiz.htm.

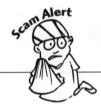

Phony HIV Tests

What kind of slime would make a buck by selling phony HIV test results? The FDA recently shut down one con artist who was selling phony HIV home-test kits. Customers paid $40 and got a coin-toss diagnosis. This crook is serving five years in jail, but there are plenty more who have taken his place online.

Testing

More than 200,000 Americans are unaware they are infected with HIV, according to the Centers for Disease Control and Prevention (CDC). What is the test, how do you find it, and what about anonymity? The Web gives you information about local health departments, private doctors, hospitals, and special sites that provide HIV testing. Many are anonymous—you are identified by a number. Others are confidential. Some go on your medical records and could be accessed by your medical insurance company, so check ahead of time if this is important to you. Be sure to get tested at a site that helps you interpret the test results and provides counseling.

A shortcut to finding a test in your area is the HIV/AIDS Testing site from the CDC (http://www.hivtest.org). This site explains and promotes early testing for those at risk. Download .pdf (readable with the Adobe Acrobat reader and available for free download online) documents about how HIV is transmitted, how to avoid getting infected, and how to get tested. Click **HIV Testing Sites** for a list of locations near you.

We advise you not to go the Internet route with home-test kits, most of which give inaccurate results, according to the Federal Trade Commission (FTC). The FTC tested a variety of Internet home test kits using known HIV-infected donors. Yet every time, the kits judged the user to be healthy. As of this writing, only one home kit for HIV has been approved by the FDA: Home Access Express HIV-1 Test System. You don't get instant results with this test—you're really only *collecting* the blood at home. You mail a drop of blood on a special card to a laboratory, and then call a hotline to learn the results from a trained counselor.

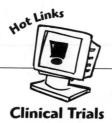

Hot Links

Clinical Trials

http://www.thebody.com/hivnews/aidscare/dec97/trials.html

Should you participate in clinical trials? Read the pros and cons and guidelines for deciding in an article from AIDS Care posted on The Body. Also check out "How Drugs Get Approved" (http://www.thebody.com/nmai/approval.html).

Treatment

Medical advances of the last few years—particularly protease inhibitors—are extending the life expectancies of people with HIV and permitting them to live active, healthy lives. If you are HIV-positive, work closely with your personal physician to determine a course of treatment that is best for you. Use the Internet to inform yourself so that your conversations with your physician are as useful as possible.

Do not, however, let the Internet play God. If you read about a treatment option that sounds better than anything your doctor has suggested, remember that adage, "If it sounds too good to be true, it probably is." Unless it comes from a respected medical journal or organization, take an announcement of a miracle treatment for AIDS for what it is: an ad, a come-on, a scam. Realize this: If there were a cure for AIDS, no reputable medical organization would hide it from you!

That doesn't mean that alternative treatments don't hold promise—they might. But let your doctor be your guide, and be sure to tell him or her what you're trying if you branch out on your own.

Before you try an alternative treatment, inform yourself about the medically accepted treatments at the HIV/AIDS Treatment Information Service site, http://www.hivatis.org/. The HIV/AIDS Treatment Information Service (ATIS) provides information about federally approved treatments and treatment guidelines, as well as publications and news releases, such as a warning about a home test that gives unreliable results (see Figure 24.1). A link to its sister site, the AIDS Clinical Trials Information Service (ACTIS), provides information about new treatments being studied in clinical trials.

Figure 24.1

Treatment information and guidelines are detailed at the HIV/ATIS site.

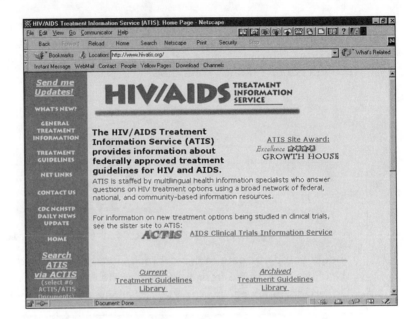

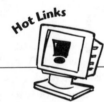

AIDS-Related Quackery and Fraud

http://www.quackwatch.com/01QuackeryRelatedTopics/aids.html

Quackbuster Stephen Barrett, M.D., debunks AIDS quack cures, immune boosters, bogus test products, and related frauds. You won't fall for the flatworm theory or aloe-juice cure after you read this.

Run, Don't Walk: Spotting Quacks

Is there no end to the AIDS scams online? Treatments, nutritional supplements, mechanical devices, drugs, and even burial fees are advertised online. Fraudulent AIDS treatment products and services cost trusting consumers $10 billion annually.

Treatment scams can hurt you in several ways:

➤ The treatment, which has not been medically tested, can make your condition even worse.

➤ Even if the "treatment" is harmless, not getting the therapy you really need can do you harm.

➤ You give up your hard-earned money to these quacks.

Many quack sites advertise cures for AIDS. First, understand that no cure exists. There are treatments that can improve your health, extend your life, and improve your quality of life and comfort, but there's no cure. If there were, the medical establishment and the media would shout it from the rooftops.

A quack AIDS treatment can be recognized by these warning signs:

➤ It claims to be a "cure."

➤ The treatment is "quick," "painless," "easy," "special," "secret," "miraculous," "ancient," or "foreign."

➤ No information indicates the product's approval or side effects.

➤ The treatment is "experimental," yet you have to pay to use it.

➤ A medical establishment or government conspiracy is withholding the "truth" from you.

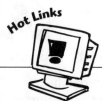

Ten Ways to Spot a Quack or Fraudulent Product

`http://www.flairs.org/tcrs/Fraud3.htm`

Use this excellent checklist from the AIDS Health Fraud Task Force (Florida) that shows you how to "investigate before you participate."

Research

If you want to know what's going on in medical research about HIV/AIDS and you're hungry for more than the news releases, but you're not ready to go straight to the medical journals, these sites can serve as your middleman.

HIV/AIDS Information Center

`http://www.ama-assn.org/special/hiv/hivhome.htm`

The *Journal of the American Medical Association* (JAMA) maintains this comprehensive site, including Newsline (updates, in-depth reports, and conference coverage), Library (the latest from the medical literature), Treatment Center (guidelines, treatment reviews, and resources), Education and Support Center (resources for patients and professionals), Prevention (facts, updates, and references), Policy (reviews, references, and resources), and Best of the Net (JAMA's reviewers' top site selections). Designed as a resource for physicians and other health professionals, this is not easy reading, but it's an up-to-date and authoritative resource.

The DIRT on AIDS

http://www.CritPath.Org/aric/dirtmain.htm

A quarterly online newsletter of Direct Information on Research and Treatment (DIRT) presented by ARIC, the AIDS Research Information Center, whose mission is "Patient Empowerment Through Information." The style is academic and tight; the information is medically accurate.

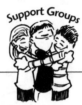

HIV Support Groups

Fighting HIV/AIDS, or caring for someone waging this war, can be easier with support. The Internet offers the comfort of "talking" to others in complete anonymity:

➤ **misc.health.aids**   This is a newsgroup for HIV/AIDS info and support.

➤ **sci.med.aids**   This is a moderated group that offers regular postings of AIDS-related magazine articles and newsletters. Postings can also be accessed through their mailing list.

➤ **http://www.thebody.com/connect.shtml**   You can find bulletin boards and chat at The Body Web site.

Start Here: HIV/AIDS Info Sites

All of our "Medical Super Sites" have extensive information about HIV/AIDS and are excellent starting points. In addition, the following sites are exceptional resources.

The Body

http://www.thebody.com

A superb AIDS and HIV resource, The Body's mission is to: "1. Use the Web to lower barriers between patients and clinicians; 2. Demystify HIV/AIDS and its treatment; 3. Improve patients' quality of life; 4. Foster community through human connection." You can read articles from the 30,000-document library, updated daily. Volunteer for clinical studies, learn about different treatments, connect to others, and get answers from experts. There's even an art gallery. This site will keep you busy for days.

HIV InSite

http://hivinsite.ucsf.edu/

This "Gateway to AIDS Knowledge" from the University of California at San Francisco AIDS Resource Institute has in-depth information about research findings, clinical trials, prevention, and social issues. Read a report about HIV/AIDS in your state or in another country. The links are diverse and plentiful. You'll find everything here.

HIV and Hepatitis.com

http://www.hivandhepatitis.com/

The aim of this site is "to improve quality of life; to slow disease progression; and to increase survival time among the hundreds of millions of people living with HIV, hepatitis B, or hepatitis C." You'll find the latest news about treatment options, vaccines, results of clinical trials, drugs, and other late-breaking reports here. You can even participate in a teleconference with medical experts who discuss treatment-related issues.

Critical Path Aids Project

http://www.critpath.org/

Founded by persons with AIDS (PWAs), this site's mission is "to provide treatment, resource, and prevention information in wide-ranging levels of detail—for researchers, service providers, treatment activists, but, first and foremost, for other PWAs who often find themselves in urgent need of information quickly and painlessly." You'll find annotated links and late-breaking news, updated daily.

HealthWeb AIDS

http://www.uic.edu/depts/lib/health/hw/aids/

This site has annotated links to dozens of selected HIV/AIDS resources. A collaboration of the Library of the Health Sciences University of Illinois at Chicago, Midwest AIDS Training and Education Center, and the HealthWeb Project.

AIDS & HIV: Alternative Medicine Resources

http://www.pitt.edu/~cbw/hiv.html

If you want to learn about alternative treatments without spending your time and money on therapies that haven't been tested, this jump site reviews sites presenting evidence-based information about alternative HIV/AIDS treatments.

The Least You Need to Know

➤ The Internet is a valuable source of up-to-date, credible, and confidential information about all aspects of HIV/AIDS.

➤ Use authoritative medical sites to learn about treatments and clinical trials.

➤ Be wary of the abundant AIDS scams on the Internet, especially any site that claims to have a cure for AIDS.

➤ Do not use the Internet as a substitute for medical attention from your physician.

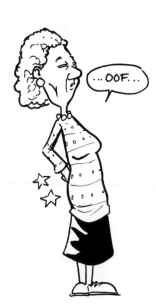

...OOF...

Chapter 25

Osteoporosis

In This Chapter

➤ Learning how osteoporosis occurs and how it affects the body

➤ Getting information about how to prevent and slow osteoporosis with lifestyle choices

➤ Learning about medications that retard bone loss

Osteoporosis means "porous bone." It is characterized by loss of bone mass, leading to increasingly fragile bones and the risk of fracture. In simpler terms, your bones get thin and brittle, and are likely to break. Fractures occur mostly in the hip, spine, and wrist. Eighty percent of people affected by osteoporosis are women.

More than 26 million persons in the United States are affected by osteoporosis, and many don't know they are losing bone. Bone loss is silent and painless—until you get a fracture.

Use this chapter to bone up on this debilitating condition by learning what it is, how to prevent it, and how to manage your life if you're living with osteoporosis.

Prevention

Your body has 206 living bones. These bones are continually building up and breaking down, a process called remodeling. Women reach their peak bone mass before they are 30, while men continue to build bone until about 35. How much peak bone mass you reach depends mainly on genetics.

As you age, the bones start to break down more than they build up. By late middle age, you probably have decreased bone density.

You can take action to keep your bones strong at any age. If you're young, don't wait until you're nearing retirement age before you start to think about protecting yourself against osteoporosis. Take preventive steps now—whatever your age—your bones need it.

The FDA recommends these preventive measures to guard against osteoporosis:

➤ Get enough calcium and vitamin D. Calcium is the main mineral in bone, and few of us get enough of it.

➤ Engage in regular physical activity, such as walking and strength training. Weight-bearing and impact activities are best to keep bones healthy, but any exercise is better than none.

➤ Don't smoke. Cigarette smoke is harmful to bone.

➤ If you drink alcohol, do so in moderation. Alcohol abuse can cause loss of calcium.

If you are an older, small-boned woman, your risk goes up. There are a number of other risk factors, so consult your physician. The following sites inform you about risk factors and what you can do to minimize your risk.

Osteoporosis: It's Never Too Late to Protect Your Bones

http://www.mayohealth.org/mayo/9711/htm/osteopor.htm

How does osteoporosis develop, who is at risk, and what can we do to prevent it? This detailed article from the Mayo Clinic answers these questions.

Bone Builders: Support Your Bones with Healthy Habits

http://vm.cfsan.fda.gov/~dms/fdbones.html

"Your body's 206 living bones continually undergo a buildup, breakdown process called remodeling." This extensive guide from the FDA examines how you can keep your bones strong, including getting enough calcium and exercising.

Exercise and Osteoporosis

http://www.mayohealth.org/mayo/9808/htm/exe_osteo.htm

The Mayo Clinic spells out what kinds of exercise work to lower the risk of osteoporosis, including an illustrated series of back exercises.

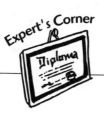

Expert's Corner

"Stronger muscles stimulate bone growth. Walking is great for cardiovascular fitness, but it has only a mild effect on bone. This can be important over time—people with a lifelong walking habit have stronger bones as a result. But walking doesn't produce the relatively rapid improvements in bone density that are seen with strength training and higher-impact activities. Strengthening exercise has another benefit of significance for people concerned about fractures: It helps improve balance, which means fewer falls. That's why it's so important to include strength training in any exercise program designed to counter osteoporosis."

—Miriam E. Nelson, Ph.D., and Sarah Wernick, authors of *Strong Women Stay Young*, *Strong Women Stay Slim* and *Strong Women, Strong Bones* (www.strongwomen.com)

Start Here: Osteoporosis Info Sites

If you've determined that you or a loved one is at risk for osteoporosis, or if you already know you have it, read as much as you can to understand the disease. The following are terrific starting places for learning the facts about osteoporosis.

Osteoporosis: What Is It?

http://www.nof.org/osteoporosis/osteoporosis.htm

This patient guide from the National Osteoporosis Foundation explains what osteoporosis is, facts and statistics, assessing your bone health, and more.

Osteoporosis

http://www.osteo.org/osteolinks.html

Get both general and specific information from this site from the National Institutes of Health, Osteoporosis, and Related Bone Diseases National Resource Center. Be sure to read **Fast Facts on Osteoporosis** and **Osteoporosis Overview**.

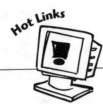

Osteoporosis: Bone Health

http://www.nof.org/osteoporosis/bonehealth.htm

It's hard to picture what happens to bones with osteoporosis, but these close-up photos clearly show the difference between normal and osteoporotic bones.

Boning Up on Osteoporosis

http://www.fda.gov/fdac/features/796_bone.html

This excellent guide from *FDA Consumer* clearly explains how osteoporosis happens, risk factors and how to prevent them, and treatment options.

Osteoporosis

http://www.intelihealth.com

Go to the More Featured Areas list at the right, and then look in the Click to See More box until you see **Osteoporosis**. (Believe me, you don't want to type the direct URL.) This site gives an extremely clear explanation of osteoporosis: symptoms, risk factors, diagnosis, and treatment.

The Osteoporosis Center

http://www.endocrineweb.com/osteoporosis/

EndocrineWeb.com presents an illustrated introduction to osteoporosis, including diagnosis, maintaining bones, exercise, calcium, and more.

Osteoporosis: Risk Factors, Screening, and Treatment

http://www.cbs.medscape.com

Type **Osteoporosis** in the Quick Search box to reach several overview articles from CBS HealthWatch and Medscape. Free registration gets you access to more in-depth information, including "what your doctor reads."

Osteoporosis@thrive

`http://www.thriveonline.com/health/osteo/index.html`

ThriveOnline hosts a large osteoporosis center with information, self-help tools, advice, and a supportive community (see Figure 25.1).

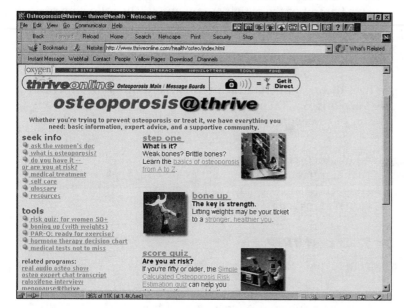

Figure 25.1

ThriveOnline's osteoporosis site offers information and support.

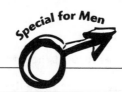

Osteoporosis in Men

`http://www.osteo.org/r603men.html`

We think of osteoporosis as a condition that affects women, but it can be a significant disease for men also, especially for men over the age of 75. This article from the National Institutes of Health, Osteoporosis, and Related Bone Diseases National Resource Center addresses the topics men want to know about how osteoporosis affects them.

Living with Osteoporosis

One in two women and one in eight men over 50 suffer fractures from osteoporosis. The first fracture is usually a wrist fracture. Hip fractures, which occur with falls, can be debilitating or even life-threatening.

If you have osteoporosis, you have several challenges: managing the disease, avoiding falls, and living an expansive life full of the activities you enjoy. The following sites can help you with these challenges.

Avoiding Falls

Thirty percent of people over the age of 65 fall each year, according to the American Academy of Orthopaedic Surgeons. 35,700 people die each year from complications from hip fractures as a result of osteoporosis, the National Osteoporosis Foundation reports.

To protect yourself against falls, incorporate balance moves into your physical activities. Take exercise classes that emphasize balance, such as Tai Chi, yoga, or other martial arts. Use my own low-impact, balance-intensive, aerobic exercise video, *The New LI Teknique* (http://www.fitnesslink.com/joanprice/litek.htm).

Don't Let a FALL Be Your Last TRIP

http://www.aaos.org/wordhtml/pat_educ/fallsbro.htm

"Falls are not natural occurrences. You can prevent falls." This guide from the American Academy of Orthopaedic Surgeons offers plenty of tips for avoiding falls, including how to fall-proof your house.

Falls: You Can Reduce Your Risk

http://www.mayohealth.org/mayo/9709/htm/falls.htm

The Mayo Clinic explains why you are more likely to fall as you get older, and what you can do to improve balance and eliminate home hazards to avoid falls.

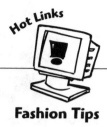

Hot Links

Fashion Tips

http://www.nof.org/patient_info/fashion_tips.htm

If you have curvature of the spine, finding clothes that fit and flatter is difficult. This site presents fashion and design tips from Beauty in All Forms, a fashion project founded by the National Osteoporosis Foundation in partnership with New York's Fashion Institute of Technology.

Treatment

It's never too late to take action to protect your bones. Get enough calcium—from 1000 to 1500 mg a day, depending on your age. Also take vitamin D, which is necessary for the body to absorb calcium. Exercise regularly, doing both weight-bearing aerobic exercise (like walking or dancing) and strength training.

Your physician may prescribe medication to help maintain bone health. The Food and Drug Administration (FDA) has approved four medications for prevention and/or treatment of osteoporosis: Estrogen replacement therapy or hormone replacement therapy (ERT/HRT), alendronate, raloxifene, and calcitonin. These medications slow or stop bone loss, increase bone density and reduce fracture risk. They don't "cure" osteoporosis.

Discuss with your doctor which treatment is best for your individual needs. Educate yourself about the medications that doctors are prescribing for osteoporosis at the following sites.

Patient Info: Medications and Osteoporosis

http://www.nof.org/patient_info/medications.htm

"Although there is no cure for osteoporosis, there are steps you can take to prevent it or to slow or stop its progress." This article describes the currently available medications that have been approved by the FDA.

Medical Treatment

http://www.thriveonline.com/health/osteo/seek.medical.html

This site from ThriveOnline describes the most common medications available today—and some you might see in the future.

315

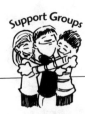

Osteoporosis Support Groups

`http://www.nof.org/patient_info/support_groups.htm`

The National Osteoporosis Foundation sponsors two kinds of osteoporosis support groups: Building Strength Together, which is a face-to-face community group, and Linking Up, which provides men and women between the ages of 20 to 50 with a list of potential pen pals or phone pals.

The Least You Need to Know

➤ You can improve the health of your bones with calcium, vitamin D, and exercise, and by quitting smoking.

➤ Reputable Web sites explain how osteoporosis occurs and what you can do to lower your risk.

➤ If you have osteoporosis, online information teaches you how to avoid falls.

➤ Educate yourself about medications for osteoporosis so that you can discuss them with your physician.

GLOSSARY

abstract   Brief summary of a research study.

allergy   The immune system reacts abnormally to a substance that is usually not harmful.

alternative/complementary medicine   A broad term covering a range of healing practices and treatments that are not generally used by physicians or hospitals and are often not reimbursed by medical insurance companies.

Alzheimer's disease   A progressive, degenerative disease that attacks the brain and results in impaired thinking, behavior, and memory.

anorexia nervosa   An eating disorder characterized by self-starvation while still seeing oneself as fat.

antidepressants   Medications used to treat depression.

arthritis   Refers to more than 100 different diseases, usually chronic, that cause pain, swelling, and limited movement in joints and connective tissue.

asthma   A chronic respiratory disease that causes a tightening of the chest and difficulty breathing due to inflammation and narrowing of the airways.

autopsy   A surgical operation performed by specially trained physicians on a dead body in order to learn the truth about the person's health and cause of death.

benign prostatic hyperplasia (BPH)   A non-cancerous enlargement of the prostate that leads to difficulty urinating.

biofeedback A treatment technique that trains people to use signals from their own bodies to improve their health.

bookmark When you bookmark a Web page, your computer saves the name and address of the site and keeps it in a file so that you can access it quickly at any time without retyping the URL.

browse Visiting one Web site after another, looking for information that might interest you.

bulimia An eating disorder characterized by binge eating followed by self-induced purging (vomiting).

cardiovascular disease Diseases that affect the heart and the blood vessels, including heart disease.

chat rooms Online areas where you can correspond in "real time" with other people who are online at the same time.

chronic Pain or condition that lasts more than six months and is likely to remain constant or recur.

dementia A medical condition in which the way the brain works is disrupted, resulting in loss of intellectual function.

depression Illness characterized by prolonged, severe, and debilitating sorrow or despair that interferes with daily life and does not get better on its own.

diabetes A disease where the body is unable to produce or respond to insulin in order to maintain proper blood glucose levels. The body either doesn't make enough insulin or can't use its own insulin efficiently, so blood sugar builds up.

dysmenorrhea Menstrual cramps.

erectile dysfunction Impotence, the inability to achieve or sustain an erection.

fibromyalgia An arthritic condition characterized by aches and pain in the joints, muscles, and tendons throughout the body, especially along the spine.

HRT Hormone replacement therapy; the use of estrogen combined with progestin to treat menopausal symptoms and prevent some long-term effects of menopause.

infertility The inability to become pregnant after one year of frequent and unprotected sexual intercourse. (Infertility is not the same thing as sterility—the inability to conceive a child under any circumstance.)

insulin The hormone that helps glucose (blood sugar) get into the cells.

jump site   A Web site that provides categorized listings of links to other sites, rather than its own content. A jump site is most useful when the sites are carefully screened by experts in the field.

link   Short for hyperlink; a reference to another document on the World Wide Web. Links are highlighted lines of text that take you to a Web site when you click them with your mouse.

mailing lists   Subscriber email mailing lists on a particular topic. You subscribe by sending your email address to a subscription address; then follow directions to send mail and receive the emails all the other subscribers sent to the list that day.

menopause   When menstruation stops permanently. A woman is said to have gone through menopause when she hasn't had a menstrual period for a year.

message boards   Also known as bulletin boards and forums, these are topic areas on Web sites where you can post messages on or read and respond to what others have written on a particular topic.

metabolic rate   The rate at which you burn calories. This varies from person to person, and is raised by physical activity and by amount of muscle mass.

osteoarthritis   Also known as degenerative joint disease, the most common type of arthritis, characterized by a breakdown of cartilage in the joints.

osteoporosis   Loss of bone mass, leading to increasingly fragile bones and the risk of fracture.

perimenopause   The years immediately preceding menopause, when symptoms have begun but menstruation has not ceased.

placebo   A drug or other preparation that has no real medicinal effect but is given for its psychological effect on the patient.

placebo effect   The effect that patients who believe a substance will work often experience when they get better although their recovery has nothing to do with what the substance contains.

prostate   The gland surrounding the urethra and immediately below the bladder in males. (Don't mispronounce it as **prostrate**, which means lying down flat on the ground.)

quackery   The promotion of a medical remedy that doesn't work or hasn't been proven to work.

rheumatoid arthritis   A type of chronic arthritis that affects joints symmetrically (on both sides of the body) and may also affect the skin, heart, lungs, nerves, blood, eyes, or kidneys. It is an autoimmune disease, unlike osteoarthritis.

search engine   A Web site that takes a word or phrase that you've typed and searches the Web for sites that relate to your query.

secure site   A Web site that keeps confidential information secure by encrypting it before transmitting it over the Internet.

self limited   Pain or injury that recovers on its own, opposite of **chronic**.

spam   Also known as "junk email," an email, bulletin board, or newsgroup message that is posted repeatedly in inappropriate places. This might include unsolicited commercial email that tries to sell you something, or derogatory messages regarding lifestyle, political views, or religion.

STDs   Sexually transmitted diseases, also known as venereal diseases, a broad term that refers to more than 50 diseases and syndromes that may be transmitted sexually, usually through the exchange of body fluids, such as semen, vaginal secretions, and blood.

stroke   A "brain attack" that occurs when blood circulation to the brain fails. It may cause death or disability.

therapeutic interaction   The effect a drug or herb can have on a disease state; usually this is an adverse effect on a medical condition other than the one for which you are taking the medication.

type 1 diabetes   Previously called insulin-dependent diabetes mellitus or juvenile-onset diabetes. The body stops producing insulin, requiring insulin injections.

type 2 diabetes   Previously called non-insulin-dependent diabetes mellitus or adult-onset diabetes. The body still produces insulin but does not use it properly.

Index

Joan Price, M.A., Helps You Get Lively and Make Good Health a Habit!

"Joan teaches even the 'exer-phobic' that exercise can be fun!"

—*Richard Simmons*

"Picture your favorite teacher, stand-up comic, and fitness maven rolled into one, and you have Joan Price."

—*convention participant*

Joan Price is a health-and-fitness writer and speaker. She educates, energizes, and entertains audiences with her books, articles, speeches, workout video, exercise classes, and personal training.

Joan Price Is Your Speaker Solution!

Is your organization planning a convention or health fair? Joan touches audiences' hearts, opens their minds, and motivates them to make changes in their lives. Whether you need a motivational speaker with a difference, or a health-and-fitness speaker to teach your group the latest facts about exercise, Joan's moving personal story, plus her entertaining, jaunty, and accessible style, will make your event memorable. Joan can also lead a variety of exercise classes for your event.

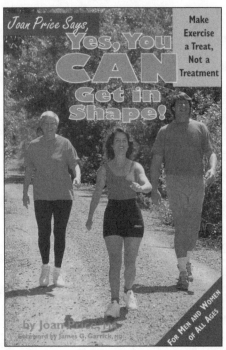

Here's How Joan Can Help You Today

If you need help getting in shape, Joan's book is for you! *Joan Price Says, Yes, You CAN Get in Shape!* helps you break through barriers and create your own fitness program—one that you'll enjoy enough to do! Learn how to stick to your shape-up resolution, even if you never did before!

Startle your muscles and your mind with *The New LI Teknique*, a revolutionary, high-intensity, low-impact aerobic exercise program incorporating the challenge of balance moves! The LI Teknique blends moves and techniques from aerobic dance, ballet, muscle conditioning, martial arts, and balance. Your exercise solution for a vigorous, safe, and sane aerobic workout!

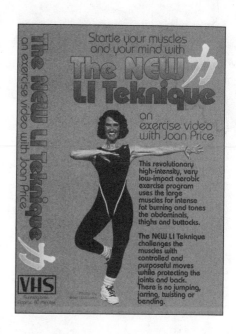

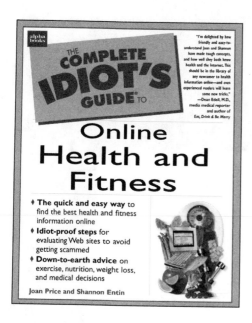

The Complete Idiot's Guide to Online Health and Fitness by Joan Price and Shannon Entin is your authoritative guidebook to the most valuable health, fitness, nutrition, and weight-loss sites on the Web. Joan and Shannon show you the best, steer you away from the worst, and teach you to tell the difference.

Also Available from Joan

Order your Dyna-Bands™—stretchy exercise-weight latex bands—and strengthen your muscles without using weights. They're simple to use, light and portable for traveling, easy to store, and nothing breaks if you drop one on your foot. Free instructions are provided.

How Can I Contact Joan Price?

Visit Joan's Web site, www.joanprice.com, email her at jprice@sonic.net, or phone toll-free 1-888-BFITTER (234-8837).